ROGI PARIKSHA
&
ROGA PARIKSHA

DIAGNOSTIC TOOLS OF AYURVEDA

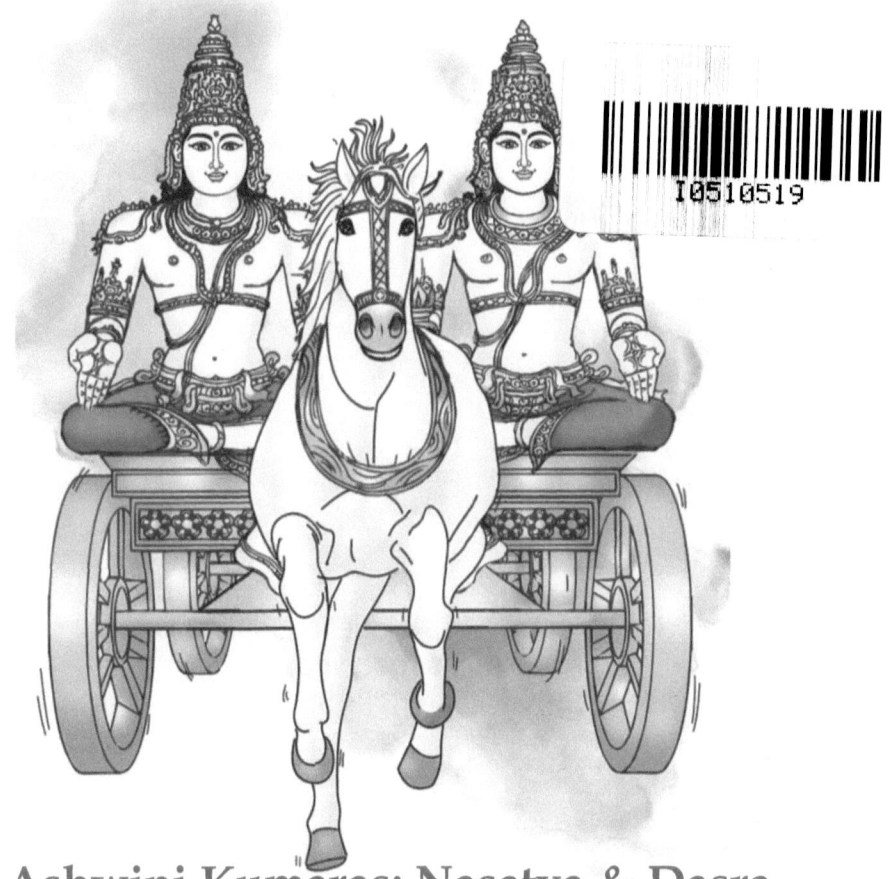

I0510519

Ashwini Kumaras: Nasatya & Dasra

Dr. Madella Gautham

Copyright © 2019 Madella Gautham
All rights reserved.
ISBN: 978-1-7013-5516-3

PREFACE

Rogi Pariksha & Roga Pariksha (Diagnostic tools of Ayurveda) is a clinical hand book with collection of Diagnostic methods from classics of Ayurveda. A Specific book to Roga Vignana and vikruti vignana department.

Dr. M. Gautham

ACKNOWLEDGEMENT

In this occasion of completion of my work, I most sincerely convey thanks with best of my respects and gratitude to my honorable Guide **Dr. K. Venkat Sivudu,** for his guidance, care and valuable suggestions throughout the course of my study have helped in completing this work successfully. His constant inspirations, encouragement, support and affection throughout the preparation of this work gave me considerable impulsion in achieving the milestone.

I avail this opportunity to express my gratitude, respect and courtesy to my Co-Guide, **Dr. Pallavi. G** and to **Dr. V. Gopala Krishnaiah,** whose harmonious help, valuable suggestions was of great help in achieving this milestone.

I am thankful to all those who have helped me directly or indirectly during this endeavour.

Dr. M. Gautham

Dedicated
To
My Wife
Dr. G. S. Rajya Lakshmi
BAMS

Index

Contents	Page No.
Pariksha	1
Roga Pariksha	1
Rogi Pariksha	1
Pariksha Prayojana	1
Different methods of Rogi & Roga Pariksha	5
Rogi Pariksha & Roga pariksha using Knowlegde of Pramanas	8
Darshanaadi Trividha Pariksha	18
Shad vidha Pariksha	18
Kaaranaadi Dasa vidha Pariksha	21
Diagramatic Representation of Ten Factors - examined before initiating Action (Chikitsa) with an example of 'Dadru Kusta.'	24
Desha Pariksha	25
Bhoomi Desha Pariksha	26
Atura Desha pariksha	27
Atura Ayu Pramana Pariksha	27
Atura Bala Dosha Pramana Pariksha / Dasa vidha Atura Pariksha	33
Prakruti	33
Vikruti	37
Saara	38
Samhanana	47
Pramana	48
Satmya	53
Satva	53
Ahaara Shakti	55
Vyayama Shakti	55
Vayah	56

Shat Kriya Kaala	59
1. Sanchaya	59
2. Prakopa	60
3. Prasara	60
4. Sthana Samshrayam	63
5. Vyakti	65
6. Bhedam	66
Nidaana Panchaka in Roga Pariksha	70
1. Nidaana	70
2. Purvarupa	71
3. Linga	73
4. Upashaya	74
5. Samprapti	78
Ashta Sthana Rogi Pariksha	82
1. Naadi	82
2. Mutra	88
3. Mala	92
4. Shabdha	94
5. Sparsha	94
6. Rupa	94
7. Drik	96
8. Jihwa	97

❀ · ❀ · ❀ · ❀ · ❀ · ❀ · ❀

Rogi Pariksha & Roga Pariksha

- **Pariksha:**

परि+ईक्ष = परीक्ष

The word 'Pariksha' derived from the root 'iksh' which means- 'to view, to consider, to examine' with the preposition 'Pari' fixed before the root which means 'from all sides'. Thus 'Pariksha' means 'viewing or examining an object from all sides'.

"परीक्ष्यते व्यवस्थाप्यते वस्तु स्वरूपमनयेति परीक्षा प्रमाणानि"

Ch.Su.11/17 Chakrapani.

Through which 'vastu swarupam' gets established is said as Pariksha or Pramana.

- **Roga:** "रुजतीति रोगः A.H.Ni.1/1. Sarvanga sundari. The one that gives pain is Roga.

- **Rogi:** "रोगी व्याधितः" A.H.Ni.1/22. Sarvanga sundari. The person afflicted with Vyadhi/Roga is Rogi.

- **Roga Pariksha** is the examination of Roga.

- **Rogi Pariksha** is the examination of Rogi.

- **Pariksha Prayojana:**

परीक्षायास्तु खलु प्रयोजनं प्रतिपत्ति ज्ञानम्| प्रतिपत्ति र्नाम यो विकारो यथा प्रतिपत्तव्यस्तस्य तथा sनुष्ठान ज्ञानम्||१३२|| Ch.vi.8/132

(प्रतिपत्तव्य इति अनुष्ठानेन योजयितव्यः - Chakrapani)

Purpose of this examination is to obtain knowledge regarding the line of treatment that should be adopted with a view to correcting the morbidity.

- o 'Pariksha' is helpful in establishing 'Siddhantha's:

सिद्धान्तो नाम स यः **परीक्षकैर्बहुविधं** परीक्ष्य हेतुभिश्च साधयित्वा

स्थाप्यते निर्णयः| Ch.vi.8/37

A demonstrated truth established after several examinations and reasonings is known as Siddhanta.

- o **Importance of Pariksha Prior to Chikitsa:**

रोगमादौ परीक्षेत ततोऽनन्तरमौषधम्|

ततः कर्म भिषक् पश्चा**ज्ज्ञानपूर्वं** समाचरेत्||२०|| Ch.su.20/20

A physician should first of all diagnose the disease and then he should select proper medicine. Thereafter, he should administer the therapy applying the knowledge of the science of medicine.

....**नापरीक्षित**मभिनिविशेत् ...   च. सू. ८ / २७

One should not indulge in any activity without proper examination.

.....**परीक्ष्य**कारिणो हि कुशला भवन्ति, यथा हि योगज्ञोऽभ्यासनित्य इष्वासो धनुरादायेषुमस्यन्नातिविप्रकृष्टे महति काये नापराधवान् भवति, सम्पादयति चेष्टकार्यं, तथा भिषक् स्वगुणसम्पन्न उपकरणवान् **वीक्ष्य** कर्मारभमाणः साध्यरोगमनपराधः सम्पादयत्येवातुरमारोग्येण; ... .

च. सू. १० / ५

Always proceed with their treatment after proper examination. As an archer having the knowledge and practice of archery throws arrows with the help of his bow and does not commit mistakes in hitting a massive body nearby and thus accomplishes his object, so a physician endowed with his own qualities and other accessories proceeding with the act of treatment after proper examination will certainly cure a curable patient without fail.

भिषजा प्राक् **परीक्ष्यैवं विकाराणां** स्वलक्षणम्|

पश्चात्कर्मसमारम्भः कार्यः साध्येषु धीमता||२१|| च. सू. १० / २१

A wise physician should examine the distinctive features of the diseases before and only then he should start his treatment about the curable diseases.

कार्यतत्त्व विशेषज्ञः प्रतिपत्तौ न मुह्यति|

अमूढः **फलमाप्नोति** यदमोहनिमित्तजम्||११|| Ch.vi.4/11

(प्रतिपत्तिः कर्मणां यथार्हतया ऽनुष्ठानम् - chakrapani.)

One who is well versed in the specific nature of the disease as well as the therapies required therefore rarely fails to act properly. It is only he who acts properly reap the results of proper action (i.e. achieves success).

ज्ञान बुद्धि प्रदीपेन यो नाविशति तत्त्ववित् [१] |

आतुरस्यान्तरात्मानं न स रोगां शिचकित्सति||१२|| Ch.vi.4/12.

(ज्ञानं शास्त्रं, तत्कृता बुद्धिः ज्ञानबुद्धिः| आविशति बुद्ध्याऽवगाहत इत्यर्थः|

अन्तरात्मानमिति वैद्यपक्षे अन्तःशरीरम् - chakrapani.)

When a physician who even if well versed in the knowledge of the disease and its treatment does not try to enter into the heart of the patient by virtue the light of his knowledge, he will not be able to treat the disease.

यस्तु **रोग मविज्ञाय** कर्माण्यारभते भिषक्|

अप्यौषधविधानज्ञस्तस्य सिद्धिर्यदृच्छया||२१|| Ch.su.20/21.

A physician who initiates treatment without proper diagnosis of the disease can accomplish the desired object only by chance (that is to say he cannot be sure of his success); the fact that he is well-acquainted with the knowledge of application of medicine does not necessarily guarantee his success.

यस्तु **रोग विशेषज्ञः** सर्व भैषज्य कोविदः|

देश काल प्रमाणज्ञस्तस्य [१] सिद्धि रसंशयम्||२२|| Ch.su.20/22

On the other hand, the physician who is well-versed in diagnosing diseases, who is proficient in the administration of medicines and who knows about the dosage of the therapy that varies from place to palce and season to season, is sure to accomplish the desired object.

केवलं विदितं यस्य शरीरं सर्वभावतः|

शारीराः सर्वरोगाश्च स कर्मसु न मुह्यति||३१|| Ch.vi.5/31

A physician who is well acquainted with all aspects of the entire body and all the diseases manifested there in will seldom commit mistake in treatment.

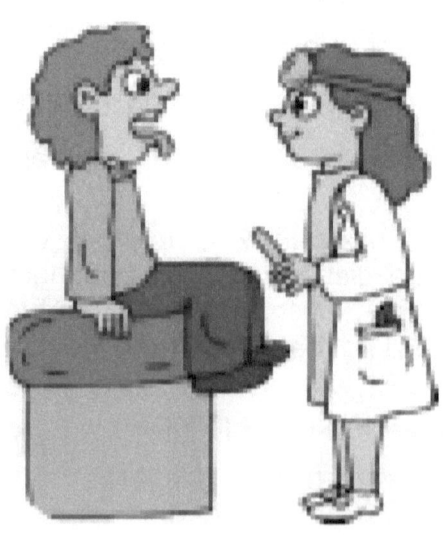

Rogi Pariksha & Roga Pariksha

Different methods of Rogi & Roga Pariksha are as:

Methods of Roga Pariksha:		Methods of Rogi Pariksha:	
Ch.Ni.1/6. A.H.Su.1/22. Y.R.Pur.1/22.	Su.Su.10/4.	Y.R.Pur.5/1	Ch.Chi.25/22. A.H.Su.1/22. Y.R.Pur.1/22.
Nidana Panchaka Pariksha	Shad vidha Pariksha	Asta Sthana Pariksha	Darshanaadi Tri vidha Pariksha
Nidana	Strotra Indriya	Naadi	Darshana
Pragrupa	Sparshana Indriya	Mutram	Sparshana
Rupa	Chakshu Indriya	Malam	Prashna
Upashaya	Rasana Indriya	Jihvaa	
Samprapti	Ghrana Indriya	Shabdam	
	Prashna	Sparsham	
		Drik	
		Akruti	

Rogi Pariksha & Roga Pariksha

Ch.Vi.4/5.	Ch.Vi.4/5.	Ch.Su.11/17.	Ch.Vi.8/79
Dwi vidha Pramana Pariksha	Tri vidha Pramana Pariksha	Chatur vidha Pramana Pariksha	Dasa vidha Pariksha
Pratyaksha	Aptopadesha	Aptopadesha	Kaarana
Anumana	Pratyaksha	Pratyaksha	Karana
	Anumana	Anumana	Kaaryayoni
		Yukti	Kaarya
			Kaaryaphala
			Anubandha
			Desha
			Kaala
			Pravrtti
			Upaya

Rogi Pariksha & Roga Pariksha

A.H.Su.12/67-68	Su.Su.35/3	Ch.Chi.30/326 Chakrapani	Ch.Vi.8/94
Dasa vidha Pariksha	Dasa vidha Pariksha	Dasa vida Pariksha	Dasa vidha Atura Pariksha
Dushyam	Vyadhi	Dosha	Prakruti
Desham	Ritu	Oushadha	Vikruti
Balam	Agni	Desha	Saara
Kaalam	Vayah	Kaala	Samhanana
Analam	Deha bala	Satmya	Pramana
Prakruti	Satva	Agni	Satmya
Vayah	Satmya	Satva	Satva
Satvam	Prakruti	Oka Satmya	Ahaara Shakti
Satmyam	Beshaja	Vayah	Vyayama Shakti
Ahaara	Desha	Bala	Vayah

Rogi Pariksha & Roga Pariksha

Rogi Pariksha & Roga Pariksha As per Charaka in describing various contexts of..			Conclusion from all the contexts as:
Ch.Su.15/17	Ch.Vi.1/3 & Ch.Vi.2/13	Ch.Si.3/6	Ch.Chi.30/326
Eka Dasa vidha Pariksha	Dwa Dasa vidha Pariksha	Nava vida Pariksha	Dasa vida Pariksha
Dosha	Dosha	Dosha	Dosha
Beshaja	Beshaja	Oushadha	Oushadha
Desha	Desha	Desha	Desha
Kaala	Kaala	Kaala	Kaala
Satmya	Satmya	Satmya	Satmya
Satva	Satva	Agni	Agni
Vayah	Vayah	Satvaadi	Satva
Bala	Bala	Vayah	Oka Satmya
Prakruti	Prakruti	Bala	Vayah
Sharira	Sharira		Bala
Ahara	Ahara		
	Saara		

Rogi Pariksha & Roga pariksha using Knowlegde of Pramanas:

Pariksha using 'Apti':

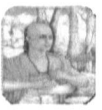

One can understand the below mentioned characteristic features of **every disease** using Aptopadesha Pramana.   Ch.Vi. 4/6.

मेवम्प्रकोपण	Prakopa	प्रकोपणं वायो रूक्षत्वादिहेतुः|	Provoking Factors of Disease Ex:- Ruksha hetu in Vata prakopa
मेवंयोनि	Yoni	योनिः वातादयः	Doshas involved in Disease
मेवमुत्थान	Uttana	उत्थानस्य उद्गमनादौ	Mode of Manifestation of Disease
मेवमात्मान	Atmaa	आत्मा स्वभावः; यथा- रोहिण्या दारुणत्वं, सन्न्यासस्य शीघ्रोपक्रमणीयत्वादि	Nature of Disease; Ex:- Darunatva of Rohini, Acuteness of Samnyasa.
मेवमधिष्ठान	Adhistaana	अधिष्ठानं शरीरमवयवा मनश्च	Location of Disease (Sharira & Manas)
मेवंवेदन	Vedana		Pain
मेवंसंस्थान	Samsthaanam	Akruti, Swarupam	Symptoms of Disease

मेवं शब्द स्पर्श रूप रस गन्ध	Shabdha Sparsha Rupa Rasa Gandha		Type of Senses felt in Disease
मेवमुपद्रव	Upadrava		Complications of Disease
मेवं वृद्धि स्थान क्षय समन्वित	Vruddi Sthana Kshaya		Aggravation, persistence, Diminution of Disease
मेवमुदर्क	Udarka	उदर्क उत्तरकालीनं फलम्	Prognosis of Disease
मेवन्नामान	Naama	-	Naming the Disease
मेवंयोगं विद्यात्	Yogam	Medications	Treatment Prescription to Disease
प्रवृत्ति	Vyadhi Pratikaara Pravrutti	ज्वरे लङ्घनपाचनाद्यर्था प्रवृत्तिः|	Ex:- Langana Pachana in Jwara
निवृत्ति	Vyadhi Pratikaara Nivrutti	निवृत्तिश्च प्रतीकारार्थी यथा- नवज्वरे दिवास्वप्नस्नानादौ	Ex:- Diva Swapna & Snana in Nava Jwara

Rogi Pariksha & Roga Pariksha

Pariksha using Pratyaksha:

One desirous of examining the specific characteristics of the health / disease by "Pratyaksha Pramana" should examine by his own senses about the objects of senses in the body of the patient except the objects related to the Tongue. Ch.Vi.4/7

Stotra Indriya Pariksha:

अन्त्रकूजनं	(gurgling sound in the intestine)
सन्धि स्फुटन मङ्गुली पर्वणां	(cracking sound in the joints including those in the fingers)
स्वर विशेषांश्च	(voice of the patient)
केचिच्छरीरोपगता: शब्दा: (कास हिक्का शब्दादय:)	other sounds in the body of the patient like (coughing and hiccup).

Chakshur Indriya Pariksha:

वर्ण	Colour
संस्थान	Shape
प्रमाण	Measurement
च्छाया:	Complexion
शरीर प्रकृति विकारौ	Natural and Unnatural states of the body
लक्षण प्रभादीनि	Signs of the Disease and Luster.

Rasana Indriya Pariksha:
using Pari-Prashna (interrogation).

Here both Praatyaksha & Anumiti are used in Rasana Pariksha.

यूकापसर्पणेन त्वस्य शरीरवैरस्यं	Moving away of Lice from the body indicates 'Sharira Vairasya.'
मक्षिकोपसर्पणेन शरीरमाधुर्यं	Attraction of flies towards the body indicates 'Sharira Madhurya.'
लोहितपित्तसन्देहे तु किं धारिलोहितं लोहितपित्तं वेति श्व काक भक्षणाद्धारि लोहित मभक्षणा ल्लोहित पित्त मित्यनुमातव्यम्,	In the case of bleeding from the body, if there is a doubt about the nature of the blood, it should be resolved by giving the blood to dogs and crows to eat. Intake of the blood by dogs and crows is indicative of its purity and rejection by these animals indicated that the blood is vitiated by pitta, i.e. the patient is suffering from raktapitta.

Ghrana Indriya Pariksha:

सर्व शरीर गतानातुरस्य प्रकृति वैकारिकान्	Normal and abonormal smells of the entire body of the patient can be examined

Sparshana Indriya Pariksha:

पाणिना प्रकृति विकृतियुक्तम्	Normal and abnormal touches of the patient can be examined by hand.

Pariksha Using Anumiti·

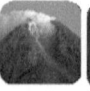

The following are the factors to be examined by inference.

Ch.Vi.4/8.

Factors to be examined are can be Understood	⇨	With the Inference of	
अग्निं	Agni	जरण शक्त्या	Pachana Shakti
बलं	Bala	व्यायाम शक्त्या	Vyayama Shakti
श्रोत्रादीनि	Stotra etc Indriyas	शब्दाद्यर्थ ग्रहणेन	Shabdadi Vishaya Grahana
मनो	Manas	sर्थाव्यभिचरणेन = Proper Knowledge of Vishaya's. The perception of specific objects even in the presence of all other senses along their respective objects. When senses and their respective objects are present together, all the sense perceptions should have occurred. Absence of such perceptions indicates that there is a third factor which determines the perception and this is mind.	
विज्ञानं	Vignanam	व्यवसायेन = Effort knowledge of a thing from proper reaction to it, e.g. when one approaches drinking water, he feels like taking water (provided, of course, he is thirsty) which indicates that he is in full knowledge of the thing along with its uses;	

रजः	Rajo Guna	सङ्गेन - नार्यादिसङ्गेन तत्कारणं रजोऽनुमीयते; rajoguna from attachment to woman etc.,-such attachments are caused by rajoguna alone;
मोह	Moha	अविज्ञानेन — Lack of understanding
क्रोध	Krodha	अभिद्रोहेण- अभिद्रोहः परपीडार्था प्रवृत्तिः ; revengeful diposition
शोकं	Shokam	दैन्येन- दैन्यं रोदनादि ; sorrowful disposition;
हर्ष	Harsha	आमोदेन - आमोदः नृत्य गीत वादित्राद्युत्सव करणम्; dancing, singing, playing musical instruments and remaining in festive mood
प्रीतिं	Preethi	तोषेण - तोषः मुख नयन प्रसादादिः; Satisfaction which is reflected by joyous appearance of the face, eyes etc. हर्षस्तु प्रीतिविशेषो मन-उद्रेक कारक इत्युक्तं भवति - Harsha is an avastha of Preethi,which causes Mano Udreka.
भयं	Bhayam	विषादेन — Depression
धैर्य	Dhairya	अविषादेन - धैर्य विपद्यपि मनसोऽदैन्यम् ; even in Vipat, Adainyata of manas or Strength of the mind even when one is in dangerous situation;
वीर्य	Viryam	उत्थानेन - उत्थानेनेति क्रियारम्भेण| - Initiating an action.

		वीर्यम् आरब्ध दुष्कर कार्येष्वव्यावृत्ति मनसः| - energy of an individual from his initiative in such actions as are normally difficult to perform.
अवस्थान	अवस्थानं स्थिर मतित्वम् - stability of the mind	अविभ्रमेण - अविभ्रमेणेति अभ्रान्त्या ; avoidance of be ing Brantha(lack of nischayata in karya).
श्रद्धा	श्रद्धाम् इच्छाम्| - Desire	अभिप्रायेण - अभिप्रायेणेति अभ्यर्थनेन| ;Requesting; ardana (wanting).
मेधां	Medha	ग्रहणेन - ग्रहणेनेति ग्रन्थादि धारणेन| - intelligence from the power of comprehension of scriptures etc.
सञ्ज्ञां	Sangnyaa-Recognising power	नाम ग्रहणेन – by the recollection of name;
स्मृतिं	मृतिमिति स्मृतिजनकं संस्कारं ; Memory	स्मरणेन - स्मरणेन हि तत्कारणं संस्कारो sनुमीयते ; -Power of Remembrance.
ह्रिय	ह्रियमिति लज्जाम् - Shyness	अपत्रपणेन - अपत्रपेणेति लज्जिता कारण ; - cause for being Shameful.
शील	शीलमिति सहजं वस्तुषु रागम्| - liking (natural liking for things)	अनुशीलनेन - अनुशीलनेनेति अनुशीलनं सन्ततशीलनं तेन; सततं यमर्थ सेवते तच्छीलोsयमित्यनुमीयते - habitual intake of things;
द्वेषं	Dvesha-	प्रतिषेधेन - प्रतिषेधेनेति व्यावृत्त्या -

	Dis liking	disinclination for accepting something;	
उपधि	उपेत्य धीयते इति उपधिः छद्म इत्यर्थः - Cheating, Deception, Fraud, Pretend, Masking	अनुबन्धेन - Subsequent manifestations तमनुबन्धेने त्युत्तरकालीन फलेन; उत्तरकालं हि भ्रात्रादि वधेन फलेन ज्ञायते- यदयमुन्मत्त च्छद्म प्रचारी चन्द्रगुप्त इति| ;-- An individual pretending to be a well wisher but actually having evil intentions can be judged from his subsequent activities like the murder of the brother etc;	
धृति	With Holding, self Command,	मलौल्येन – Steadiness, consistency, firmness	
वश्यतां	Vashyata	विधेयतया	Being Obedient
वयो भक्ति सात्म्य व्याधि समुत्थानानि	Vayah Bhakti(Iccha) Vyadhi Nidana	काल देशोपशय वेदना विशेषेण; - stage of the life, habitat, conduciveness and characteristic features of pain respectively. Age of the patient can be determined by the stage of his life, viz childhood etc. habitat of an individual determines his liking e.g. if an individual has liking for wheat and masa (phaseolus radiatus Linn.) then he should be inferred to be an inhabitant of madhyadesa (central region of the country). When something is conducive to the individual, it should be treated as wholesome. If somebody is suffering from hyperpyrexia, it can be safely inferred that the etiological factors of	

		fever are responsible for this condition.
गूढ लिङ्गं	Gooda Lingam	व्याधि मुपशयानुपशयाभ्यां - Upashaya & Anupashaya
दोष प्रमाण विशेष	Dosha Pramana	अपचार विशेषेण – Provocating Factors. अपचारविशेषणेति महताऽपचारेण भूरिदोषो भवति, स्वल्पेण स्वल्प इति| ; - When these provocative factors are in abundance, there is excessive vitiation of dosas on the other hand, if there is less of provocative factors then the vitiatin of dosas is mild;
आयुषः क्षय	Ayu Kshaya	अरिष्टैः Arista
उपस्थित श्रेयस्त्वं	Approaching prosperity (Shreya)	कल्याणाभिनिवेशन - कल्याणाभिनिवेशनेति श्रेयस्कर मार्गानुष्ठानेन ;एतद्धि अचिर भावि श्रेयसामेव भवति - Initiation of useful work
अमलं सत्त्व	Pure Satva सत्त्वमिति सत्त्वगुणोद्रेकम्	अविकारेण - अविकारेणेति रागद्वेष विकाराभावेन ; - Abhava of Raga Dwesha vikara's.
1. ग्रहण्यास्तु मृदुदारुणत्वं : The costiveness or laxity of grahani (lit. duodenum and small intestine but contextually meaning	(1-5)are known by आतुर परिप्रश्नेन - interrogating the patient.	

bowels)	
2. स्वप्न दर्शन - dreams	
3. अभिप्रायं ;अभिप्रायः भोजनादीच्छा -desires for food etc.	
4. द्विष्टेष्ट ; द्विष्टेष्टशब्देन तु द्विष्टेप्सितप्रेष्यादिग्रहणम्| - likes and dislikes	
5. सुख दुःखानि : happiness and unhappiness etc.	

Pariksha using Yukti:

The following are the examples of Yukti Pariksha.

Ch.Su.23-25.

Growth of crops:-	The combination of irrigation, ploughed land, seed and seasons.
Formation of embryo:-	The combination of six dhatus (five mahabhutas and atman).
Production of fire:-	The combination of the lower-fire-drill, upper-fire-drill and the act of drilling.
Cure of diseases:-	Fourfold efficient therapeutic measures.

Rogi Pariksha & Roga Pariksha

Darshanaadi Trividha Pariksha: Ch.Chi.25/22.

Darshana Pariksha	Sparshana Pariksha	Prashna Pariksha
1. Vayah	1. Mardava	1. Hetu
2. Varna	2. Kathina	2. Arthi - Pain
3. Sharira	3. Shaitya	3. Satmyam
4. Indriyas	4. Ushna	4. Agni Balam

Shad vidha Pariksha: Su.Su.10/4.

Stortra Indriya Pariksha:	Sparshana Indriya Pariksha:	Chakshu Indriya Pariksha	Rasana Indriya Pariksha	Ghrana Indriya Pariksha
'तत्र सफेनं रक्त मीरयन्ननिलः सशब्दो निर्गच्छति'on description of wound and its discharge such as – 'there vayu, impelling frothy blood, comes out with sound. Etc.	Sita, Ushna, Slakshna, Karkasha, Mridu, Kathinatva, Etc.	Sharira Upachaya - development of physique; Sharira Apachaya; Lakshanas of Ayu; Bala; Varna Vikara; Etc.	in prameha etc. the tastes sweet etc. are inferred by movement of flies, ants etc. and as such rasanendriya here means the gustatory organ of flies etc. and not of physician.	different types of smells in relation to 1. Arista Linga's, 2. Vrana Vyadhi's, other vyadhi's.

Prashna Pariksha:

Desam - स्त्रिविधो जाङ्गलानूप साधारण भेदात्।	Vedana Samuchra = Aggravation of Pain
Kaalam - कालो द्विविधो नित्यग आवस्थिकश्च; नित्यगः ऋतुलक्षणः; आवस्थिको द्विविधः-स्वस्थस्य बाल्यादिभेदेन, व्याधितस्य ज्वरारम्भादिकालावस्थया च।	Kaala Prakarsha – time of disesase manifestation, Etc.
Jaati – ब्राह्मणादिषु	Antar Agni : समो विषमो मन्दो
Satmya- A. Chesta Satmya काय वाङ्मनो भेदात्रि विधम् B. Ahaara Satmya on Shad vida rasa	Pravrutti & Apravrutti of 1. Vaata 2. Mutra 3. Purisha etc.आर्तवाधोगतरक्तपित्त
Atamka Samutpatti = Vyadhi Nidana	Balam

Other unmentioned diseases may be diagnosed on the basis of the symptoms of similar dosas using Shad vidha Pariksha as follows:

Vata Dosha Pariksha			Su.Su.10/5 Dalhana.			
Stortra Indriya Pariksha	Sparshana Indriya Pariksha	Chakshu Indriya Pariksha	Rasana Indriya Pariksha	Ghrana Indriya Pariksha	Prashna Pariksha
व्रणे सशब्द फेन रक्तानिला दिनिर्गमनं	पारुष्य रौक्ष्यादिकं	भस्मकपो तास्थि सवर्णत्वं	कषाय रसत्वं	कटु गन्ध लाजगन्धा दित्वं	तोदन भेदन च्छेदनादि वेदना विशेषाः

Pitta Dosha Pariksha					Su.Su.10/5 Dalhana.
Stortra Indriya Pariksha	Sparshana Indriya Pariksha	Chakshu Indriya Pariksha	Rasana Indriya Pariksha	Ghrana Indriya Pariksha	Prashna Pariksha
	श्वयथु व्रणादीनामौष्ण्यं	नील पीत वर्णत्वं	कट्वम्लर सत्वं	तीक्ष्णातसी गन्धत्वं	ओषचोष परिदाहादि का वेदना विशेषाः

Kapha Dosha Pariksha					Su.Su.10/5 Dalhana.
Stortra Indriya Pariksha	Sparshana Indriya Pariksha	Chakshu Indriya Pariksha	Rasana Indriya Pariksha	Ghrana Indriya Pariksha	Prashna Pariksha
	स्निग्धपैच्छिल्यादिकं	श्वेतत्वं	माधुर्यादि	विस्रगन्धादित्वं	कण्डूगुरुत्वादिवेदनाविशेषाः

Kaaranaadi Dasa vida Pariksha:

Examination of the following Ten Factors before initiating the Treatment. Ch.Vi.8/79.

Kaarana	तद् यत् करोति	हेतुः, कर्ता	who initiates action	Bhishak
Karana	स्तद् यदुपकरणाय उपकल्पते कर्तुः कार्याभिनिर्वृत्तौ	an instrument	which helps an agent in the performance of his action.	Bheshajam
Kaarya yoni	सा या विक्रियमाणा कार्यत्वमापद्यते	source of an action	one which becomes an action(Karya) by the process of transformation.	Dathu Vaishamyam
Kaarya	तद्यस्याभिनिर्वृत्तिमभिसन्धाय कर्ता प्रवर्तते	Action	the act by which the agent proceeds to reach the objective.	Dathu Samyam

Kaarya phala	स्तद् यत्प्रयोजना कार्याभिनिर्वृत्ति रिष्यते	Objective to reach or The object of Action.	The Object or Benifit, about which the action is initiated.	Sukha Prapti or Arogya Prapti.
Anubandha	स यः कर्तारमवश्य मनुबध्नाति कार्यादुत्तरकालं कार्यनिमित्तः शुभो वाऽप्यशुभो भावः	A compulsory Aftereffect on Kartha.	An aftereffect- good or bad- is the one which is bound (sure) to leave its impact on the agent after he has performed his action.	Ayu of Atura depends on Bhishak's Aftereffect of Karya.
Desha	देशस्त्वधिष्ठानम् ।	Site of Action	the site favourable or unfavourable to an action.	Bhumi desha & Atura desha
Kaala	कालः पुनः परिणामः	Transformation process	a process of transformation into Ritu,Ayana etc.	Samvatsara or Atura avastha

Pravrtti	प्रवृत्तिस्तु खलु चेष्टा कार्यार्था; सैव क्रिया, कर्म, यत्नः, कार्यसमारम्भश्च	The Act to obtain Karya.	The initiation of action as a means to the accomplishment of an object. This is Kriya, Karma, Effort to begin.	Prati-Karma = Chikitsa.
Upaya	उपायः पुनस्त्रयाणां कारणादीनां सौष्ठवमभिविधानं च सम्यक् कार्य कार्यफलानुबन्धव ज्यांनां, कार्याणा मभिनिर्वर्तक इत्यतस्तूपायः	Approach/ Stratergy/ Application/ Solution/ Way/ remedy / Trick / means of Action.	That which brings about excellence in the Kaarana, the Karana and the Karya yoni and their proper setting is Upaya. Such an upaya accomplishes Karya.	Excellence of the physician etc. & the Right approach of the therapy.

Diagramatic Representation of Ten Factors - examined before initiating Action (Chikitsa) with an example of 'Dadru Kusta.'

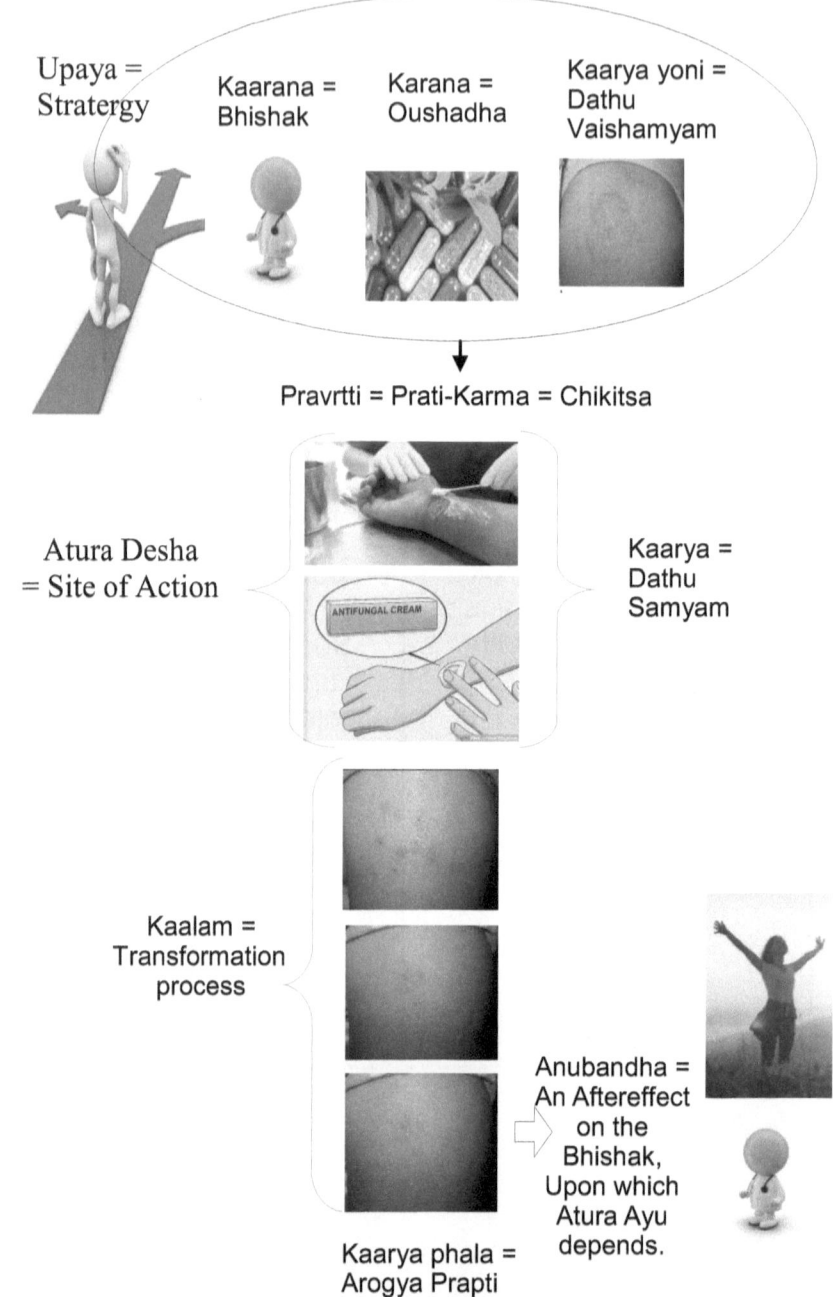

Upaya = Stratergy

Kaarana = Bhishak

Karana = Oushadha

Kaarya yoni = Dathu Vaishamyam

Pravrtti = Prati-Karma = Chikitsa

Atura Desha = Site of Action

Kaarya = Dathu Samyam

ANTIFUNGAL CREAM

Kaalam = Transformation process

Anubandha = An Aftereffect on the Bhishak, Upon which Atura Ayu depends.

Kaarya phala = Arogya Prapti

Desha Pariksha: is of 2 ways.	Ch.Vi.8/92.
Bhoomi Desha Pariksha	**Atura** Desha Pariksha / Karya Desha Pariksha
1. आतुर परिज्ञान हेतोर्वा - Provides **Atura** Parignana	1. आयुषः प्रमाण ज्ञान हेतोर्वा - Provides **Atura Ayu** Pramana gnana.
2. दौषध परिज्ञान हेतोर्वा| - Provides **Oushadha** Parignana	2. बल दोष प्रमाण ज्ञान हेतोर्वा - Provides **Atura Bala Dosha** Pramana gnana. I; e. a) Atura **Deha Bala** Pramana gnana. & b) Atura **Dosha Bala** Pramana gnana. (दोष प्रमाणानुरूपो हि भेषज प्रमाण विकल्पो बल प्रमाण विशेषापेक्षो भवति| Beshaja Pramana & Bheshaja Vikalpa depends on Atura Dosha Bala Pramana rupa & also specially on Atura Bala Pramana.)

Bhoomi Desha Pariksha for Atura Parignana:

Factors help in Atura parignana:	
कस्मिन् भूमिदेशे	जातः
	संवृद्धो
	व्याधितो
तस्मिंश्च भूमिदेशे	मनुष्याणामिदमाहारजातम्,
	इदं विहारजातम्,
	इदमाचारजातम्,
	एतावच्च बलम्,
	एवंविधं सत्त्वम्,
	एवंविधं सात्म्यम्,
	एवंविधो दोषः,
	भक्तिरियम्,
	इमे व्याधयः,
	हितमिदम्,
	अहितमिदमिति

Atura Desha Pariksha:

1. Atura Ayu Pramana Pariksha:

आयुषः प्रमाणज्ञानहेतोः पुनरिन्द्रियेषु [१] जातिसूत्रीये च

लक्षणान्युपदेक्ष्यन्ते   Ch.Vi.8/124.

It is said in form of 'Ayu Lakshana's' in Indriya Sthana & in Jati Sutriya Adhyaaya of Sharira Sthana.

The following factors should be examined by the physician desirous of ascertaining the residual span of life of the patient by direct observation, inference and scriptural testimony: Ch.Indriya.1/3.

वर्णश्च	1. Complexion	(आचारः शास्त्र शिक्षाकृतो व्यवहारः।)	
स्वरश्च	2. Voice		
गन्धश्च	3. Smell		
रसश्च	4. Taste		
स्पर्शश्च	5. Touch	स्मृतिश्च	16.memory
चक्षुश्च	6. Eyes	आकृतिश्च	17.shape
श्रोत्रंच	7. Ears	प्रकृतिश्च	18.nature
घ्राणंच	8.nose	विकृतिश्च	19. Morbidity
रसनंच	9. Tongue	बलंच	20.strength
स्पर्शनंच	10. Skin	ग्लानिश्च	21. exhaustion
सत्त्वंच	11. Mind	मेधाच	22. Intelligence
भक्तिश्च (इच्छा)	12. Desire	हर्षश्च	23. Exhileration
शौचंच	13.purity	रौक्ष्यंच	24.dryness
शीलंच (शीलं सहजं वृत्तम्)	14.conduct	स्नेहश्च	25.unctuousness
आचारश्च	15.refined behaviour	तन्द्राच	26.drowsiness (sleep)
		आरम्भश्च	27.onset

गौरवंच	28.heaviness	उपद्रवाश्च	Complication
लाघवंच	29.lightness	च्छायाच	40. Lustre
गुणाश्च	30.attributes	प्रतिच्छायाच	41. Shadow
आहारश्च	31.diet	स्वप्नदर्शनंच	42. Dream
विहारश्च	32. Regimens	दूताधिकारश्च	43.messenger
आहारपरिणामश्च	33.digestion of food	पथिच उत्पातिकंच	44.bad omens visualized by the physician on his way to the patient's house
उपायश्च	34.manifestation of the disease		
अपायश्च	35.disappearance of the disease		
व्याधिश्च	36. Characteristic features of the disease	आतुरकुले भावावस्थान्तराणिच	45. Bad omens at the residence of the patient
व्याधिपूर्वरूपंच	37.premonitory signs of the disease	भेषजसंवृत्तिश्च	46.administration of proper medicine
वेदनाश्च	38. Pain	भेषजविकारयुक्तिश्चेति	47. Effect of medicine in disease.
	39.		

After Namakarana, proceed to Kumara Pariksha which gives 'Ayu Pramana Gnana.' Ch.Sa.8/51

The following are the Deergha Ayu Lakshan's of Kumara:

एकैकजा मृदवोऽल्पाः स्निग्धाः सुबद्धमूलाः कृष्णाः केशाः प्रशस्यन्ते	1. Hair	Discrete soft, sparse, unctuous, firmly rooted and black
स्थिरा बहला त्वक्	2. Skin	Thick and not loose
प्रकृत्याऽतिसम्पन्नमीषत्प्रमाणातिवृत्तमनुरूपमातपत्रोपमं शिरः	3. Head	Constitutionally of excellent type, slightly bigger in size (than the measurement furnished in vimana 8:117), proportionate with other parts of the body and resembling an umbrella in shape
व्यूढं दृढं समं सुश्लिष्टशङ्खसन्ध्यूर्ध्वव्यञ्जनसम्पन्नमुपचितं वलिभमर्ध चन्द्राकृति ललाटं	4. Fore-Head	Broad, strong, even, compact having firm union with temporal bones, having three transverse lines, plump, having wrinkles and having the shape of a half moon
बहलौ विपुलसमपीठौ समौ नीचैर्वृद्धौ पृष्ठतोऽवनतौ सुश्लिष्टकर्णपुत्रकौ महाच्छिद्रौ कर्णौ	5. Ears	Thick, large in size, having even lobes, equal in size, having elongations downwards, bent towards back side, having compact tragus and having a big earhole.
ईषत्प्रलम्बिन्यावसङ्गते समे संहते महत्यौ भ्रुवौ	6.Eye Brows	Slightly hanging downwards separated from each other, equal in size, compact and large in size.

समे समाहितदर्शने व्यक्तभागविभागे बलवती तेजसोपपन्ने स्वङ्गापाङ्गे चक्षुषी	7. Eyes	Equal in size, having fixed look, having clear cut divisions (of pupil, iris or black portion of the eye, sclera or white portion of the eye) strong, lustrous, beautiful and having beautiful apanga (corners of eyes)
ऋज्वी महोच्छवासा वंशसम्पन्नेषदवनता ग्रा नासिका	8. Nose	Straight, capable of taking deep breath well ridged, and slightly curved at the tip
महद्जुसुनिविष्टदन्त मास्यम्	9. Mouth	Big in size straight and having (two rows of)compact teeth
आयामविस्तारोपप न्ना श्लक्ष्णा तन्वी प्रकृतिवर्णयुक्ता जिह्वा	10 . Tongue	Having proper length and breadth, smooth thin and endowed with natural colour
श्लक्ष्णं युक्तोपचयमूष्मोपप न्नं रक्तं तालु	11. Palate	Smooth plump, hot in touch and red in colour
महानदीनः स्निग्धो sनुनादी गम्भीर समुत्थो धीरः स्वरः	12. Voice	Profound, not sluggish sweet, having echo, deep toned and steady
नातिस्थूलौ नातिकृशौ विस्तारोपपन्नावास्य प्रच्छादनौ रक्तावोष्ठौ	13. Lips	Neither very thick nor very thin, having adequate width, capable of covering the mouth cavity and red in colour
महत्यौ हनू	14. Jaws	Large in size
वृत्ता नातिमहती ग्रीवा	15. Neck	Round in shape and not very large in size

व्यूढमुपचितमुरः	16. Chest	Broad and plumpy
गूढं जत्रु पृष्ठवंशश्च	17. Clavicles And Vertiberal Column	Not visible
विप्रकृष्टान्तरौ स्तनौ	18. Breasts	Having wide space in between them
असम्पातिनी स्थिरे पार्श्वे	19. Parsva (Sides Of The Chest)	Absence of any uneven appearance downwards and firm
वृत्तपरिपूर्णायतौ बाहू सक्थिनी अङ्गुलयश्च	20. Arms, Thighs, Fingers Including Toes	Round, full and extended
महदुपचितं पाणिपादं	21. Hands And Legs	Large in size and plump.
स्थिरा वृत्ताः स्निग्धा स्ताम्रास्तुङ्गाः कूर्माकाराः करजाः	22.Nails	Firm, round, unctuous, coppery coloured, properly elevated and convex like the back of a tortoise
प्रदक्षिणावर्ता सोत्सङ्गा च नाभिः	23. Umbilicus	Whirled clock-wise and well depressed
उरस्त्रिभागहीना समा समुपचितमांसा कटी	24. Waist	Less than ¾ th of the chest in circumference, even and plump with muscles
वृत्तौ स्थिरोपचितमांसौ नात्युन्नतौ नात्यवनतौ स्फिचौ	25. Buttocks	Round firm, plump with muscles and neither excessively elevated nor excessively depressed
अनुपूर्वं वृत्तावुपचययुक्तावूरू	26. Thighs	Tapering downwards, round and plump

नात्युपचिते नात्यपचिते एणीपदे प्रगूढसिरास्थिसन्धी जङ्घे	27. Calf Region	Neither excessive plump nor excessively emaciated, having resemblance with that of a deer and having vessels, bones and joints well covered
नात्युपचितौ नात्यपचितौ गुल्फौ	28. Ankles	Neither excessively plump nor excessively emaciated
पूर्वोपदिष्टगुणौ पादौ कूर्माकारौ	29. Feet	Having the characteristic features described above and having the shape like that of a tortoise.
प्रकृतियुक्तानि वातमूत्रपुरीषगुह्यानि तथा स्वप्रजागरणायासस्मितरुदितस्तन ग्रहणानि यच्च किञ्चिदन्यदप्यनुक्तमस्ति तदपि सर्वं प्रकृतिसम्पन्नमिष्टं. विपरीतं पुनरनिष्टम्। इति दीर्घायुर्लक्षणानि		Normal flatus, urine, stool, anus, sleep, vigil,, fatigue, smiling, crying, suckling of milk and whatever else has been left unmentioned here, if conforming to what is excellent in nature, should be regarded as desirable, what is contrary to this is to be considered undesirable.

Atura Desha Pariksha:

2. Atura Bala Dosha Pramana Pariksha / Dasa vidha Atura Pariksha. Ch.Vi.8/94.

Prakruti:
Vikruti:–
Saar:-
Samhanana
Pramana
Satmya
Satva
Ahaara Shakti
Vyayama Shakti
Vayah

Prakruti Pariksha:

Prakruti :

It is the Swabhavam. Prakruti of Garbha sharia can be known by the dominance of doshas, which depend on the following factors:

1. शुक्र शोणित प्रकृतिं, sperm and ovum;

2. काल गर्भाशय प्रकृतिं, season and condition of the uterus;

3. मातुराहार विहार प्रकृतिं, food and regimens of the mother; and

4. महाभूत विकार प्रकृतिं, nature of the mahabhutas comprising the foetus.

Such Prakruti can be :
1. Sleshmala
2. Pittala
3. Vaatala
4. Samsrista – Combination of 2 doshas
5. Sama Dathava – Equilibrium of 3 doshas

Sleshma Prakruti Lakshana's :		
Gunas:	**Manifestation of Gunas in the Sharira:**	**Prakruti rupam is seen as:**
स्निग्ध	तस्य स्नेहाच्छ्लेष्मलाः स्निग्धाङ्गाः	बलवन्तो
श्लक्ष्ण	श्लक्ष्णत्वाच्छ्लक्ष्णाङ्गाः	वसुमन्तो
मृदु	मृदुत्वाद्दृष्टिसुख सुकुमारावदातगात्राः(avadaata=clear)	विद्यावन्त
मधुर	माधुर्यात् प्रभूत शुक्र व्यवायापत्याः	ओजस्विनः
सार	सारत्वात् सार संहत स्थिर शरीराः	शान्ता
सान्द्र	सान्द्रत्वादुपचित परिपूर्ण सर्वाङ्गाः	आयुष्मन्तश्च
मन्द	मन्दत्वान्मन्द चेष्टाहार व्याहाराः (vyaahaara = Speech)	
स्तिमित	स्तैमित्यादशीघ्रारम्भ क्षोभ विकाराः	
गुरु	गुरुत्वात् साराधिष्ठितावस्थित गतयः (सारगतयो न स्खलन्ति, अधिष्ठितगतयः सर्वेण पदेन महीमाक्रामन्ति, अवस्थितगतय इति अवस्थितत्वेन न चपला गतिर्भवति)	
शीत	शैत्यादल्प क्षुत्तृष्णा सन्ताप स्वेद दोषाः	
विज्जल	विज्जलत्वात् सुश्लिष्ट सार सन्धि बन्धनाः (vijjala =Picchila), (Sushlishta = properly joined)	
अच्छः	तथा sच्छत्वात् प्रसन्न दर्शनाननाः प्रसन्न स्निग्ध वर्ण स्वराश्च भवन्ति	

Pitta Prakruti Lakshana's :		
Gunas:	Manifestation of Gunas in the Sharira:	Prakruti rupam is seen as:
मुष्णं	तस्यौष्ण्यात् पित्तला भवन्त्युष्णासहा	मध्यबला
	उष्णमुखाः	मध्यायुषो
	सुकुमारावदातगात्राः	मध्यज्ञान
	प्रभूत विप्लु व्यङ्ग तिल पिडकाः	विज्ञान
	क्षुत्पिपासावन्तः	वित्तो
	क्षिप्र वली पलित खालित्य दोषाः	उपकरणवन्तश्च
	प्रायो मृद्वल्प कपिल श्मश्रु लोम केशाश्च;	
तीक्ष्णं	तैक्ष्ण्यात्तीक्ष्णपराक्रमाः	
	तीक्ष्णाग्नयः	
	प्रभूताशनपानाः	
	क्लेशासहिष्णवो	
	दन्दशूकाः (दन्दशूकाः पुनः पुनर्भक्षण शीलाः)	
द्रवं	द्रवत्वाच्छिथिलमृदुसन्धिमांसाः	
	प्रभूतसृष्टस्वेदमूत्रपुरीषाश्च;	
विस्र	विस्रत्वात् प्रभूतपूतिकक्षास्यशिरःशरीरगन्धाः;	
मम्लं कटुकञ्च	कट्वम्लत्वादल्पशुक्र व्यवायापत्याः	

Vata Prakruti Lakshana's :		
Gunas:	**Manifestation of Gunas in the Sharira:**	**Prakruti rupam is seen as:**
रूक्ष	तस्य रौक्ष्याद्वातला रूक्षापचिताल्प शरीराः प्रतत रूक्ष क्षाम सन्न सक्त जर्जर स्वरा (प्रततः प्रसृतः; सन्नः हीनः; सक्तः बद्धः; जर्जरः भग्न पात्र ध्वनि समः) or ('प्रततः प्रभूतः') जागरूकाश्च	प्रायेणाल्प बला श्चाल्पायुष श्चाल्पापत्या श्चाल्प साधना श्चाल्प धना
लघु	लघुत्वाल्लघु चपल गति चेष्टाहार व्याहाराः	
चल	चलत्वादनवस्थित सन्ध्यक्षि भ्रू हन्वोष्ठ जिह्वा शिरः स्कन्ध पाणि पादाः	
बहु	बहुत्वाद्बहु प्रलाप, कण्डरा, सिरा, प्रतानाः	
शीघ्र	शीघ्रत्वाच्छीघ्र क्षोभ शीघ्र राग विरागाः समारम्भ विकाराः त्रास श्रुत ग्राहिणो sल्प स्मृतयश्च	
शीत	शैत्याच्छीतासहिष्णवः प्रतत शीतकोद्वेपक स्तम्भाः	
परुष	पारुष्यात् परुष केश श्मश्रु रोम नख दशन वदन पाणि पादाः	
विशदः	वैशद्यात् स्फुटिताङ्गावयवाः सतत सन्धि शब्दगामि'नश्च	

Among the 3 Prakruti's:

Kaphaja Prakruti or Sama Prakruti – is with Uttama Bala & Deergha Ayu.

Heena Prakruti - is with Hina Bala & Alpa Ayu.

Vikruthi Pariksha:

विकृतिरुच्यते विकारः|

Without knowing about the **'Hetvaadi Bala'** Visesha, it is not possible to obtain Vyadhi Bala Visesha.

Vikara Pariksha based on Lakshana's of following:

Features in Rogi with respect to Roga:			Based on Resemblance of Features		
	Observe the following in the Rogi	Features of Roga said in text	Classification of Vyadhi Bala is done		
			Balavaan	Madya Bala	Alpa Bala
हेतु	हेतु	हेतु	Most of them Resemble + Mahat Hetu & Linga	Few of them Resemble + Madya Hetu & Linga	Donot Resemblance + Alpa Hetu & Linga
दोष	दोष	दोष			
दूष्य	दूष्य	दूष्य			
प्रकृति	प्रकृति	प्रकृति			
देश	देश	देश			
काल	काल	काल			
बल	बल	बल			

If the above said Doshadi of the Rogi resemble with that of the Roga & is with 'mahat' Hetu & Linga balam. Such a Roga is said to be 'Balavaan'.

If otherwise, it is 'Alpa Bala.'

If the few among the above said Doshadi of the Rogi resemble with that of the Roga & is with 'Madyama' Hetu & Linga balam. Such a Roga is said to be 'Madya Bala.'

Saara Pariksha: Ch.Vi.8/102-115.

न शरीर मात्र दर्शनादेव भिषङ्मुह्येदयमुपचितत्वाद्बलवान्, अयमल्पबलः कृशत्वात्.

It is not correct to consider just only by 'Darshana' of the 'Sharira', that

1. Balavaan due to Upachitatvaad (Sthoolatvaat) or Maha Sharira (Ati Pramana).
2. Alpa bala due to Krishatvaat / Alpa Sharira.

Some have Alpa Sharira and Krishatva yet are Balavanta.

'तत्र पिपीलिकाभारहरणवत् सिद्धिः' - पिपीलिकाभारहरणवदिति स्वल्पाः पिपीलिका यथा सारशरीरत्वेन महान्तं भारं नयन्ति, तथाऽल्पकृशशरीरा इत्यर्थः

They are like ants who have a small body and look emaciated but can carry too heavy load.

Hence Pariksha should be done based on 'Saara.'

सारशब्देन विशुद्धतरो धातुरुच्यते
साराण्यष्टौ पुरुषाणां बल मान विशेष ज्ञानार्थ मुपदिश्यन्ते
तद्यथा- त्वग्रक्त मांस मेदो ऽस्थि मज्ज शुक्र सत्त्वानीति||१०२||

Use of Saara Pariksha:

'Bala Maana Visesha Gyanartham.'

1. Twak Saara Pariksha:

Lakshana's of Twak Saara:	It Indicates:
स्निग्ध	
श्लक्ष्ण	सुख
	सौभाग्य
मृदु	ऐश्वर्य
प्रसन्न	उपभोग
सूक्ष्म · लोमा = hair	बुद्धि
अल्प · लोमा = hair	विद्या
गम्भीर · लोमा = hair	आरोग्य
सुकुमार · लोमा = hair	प्रहर्षणा
	आयुष्यत्वं
(gambhira = Deep roorted)	
सप्रभेव = Lustrous Skin	

2. Rakta Saaara Pariksha:

Lakshana's of Rakta Saara:		It Indicates:
	कर्ण	
	अक्षि	सुख
	मुख	उद्धतां (prashasta swabhava)
स्निग्ध	जिह्वा	मेधां
रक्त वर्ण	नासा	मनस्वित्वं / cheerful
श्रीमद् (श्रीमदिति शोभा युक्तम्) ?	ओष्ठ	सौकुमार्यं
	पाणि	अनतिबलं
भ्राजिष्णु (tejaswi / lustrous)	पादतल	अक्लेश सहिष्णुत्वं
	नख	उष्ण असहिष्णुत्वं
	ललाट	
	मेहनं	

3. Mamsa Saara Pariksha:

Lakshana's of Mamsa Saara:		It Indicates:
स्थिर गुरु शुभ ? मांसोपचिता	शङ्ख ललाट कृकाटिका (nape) अक्षि गण्ड हनु ग्रीवा स्कन्धो उदर कक्ष वक्षः पाणि पाद सन्धयः	क्षमां धृतिं अलौल्यं (achapalata) ? वित्तं विद्यां सुखं आर्जवं (frankness) ? आरोग्यं बलं आयुश्च दीर्घम्

4. Medo Saara Pariksha:

Lakshana's of Medo Saara:		It Indicates:
विशेषतः स्नेहो ⇨	वर्ण	
	स्वर	वित्त
	नेत्र	ऐश्वर्य
	केश	सुख
	लोम	उपभोग
	नख	प्रदानानि (charitable)
	दन्त	आर्जवं ?
	ओष्ठ	सुकुमारो
	मूत्र	उपचारतां ?
	पुरीषेषु	

5. Asthi Saara Pariksha:

Lakshana's of Asthi Saara:		It Indicates:
स्थूलाः ⇨	पार्ष्णि (heels)	
	गुल्फ (ankle)	
	जानु (knee)	महोत्साहाः
	अरत्नि (fore arm)	क्रियावन्तः
	(अरत्निः कफोणिका ?)	क्लेशसहाः
	जत्रु	सार स्थिर शरीरा
	चिबुक	आयुष्मन्तश्च
	शिरः	
	पर्व (joints) parva ?	
	अस्थि(bones)	
	नख	
	दन्त	

6. Majja Saara Pariksha:

Lakshana's of Majja Saara:		It Indicates:
मृद्वङ्गा		दीर्घायुषो
बलवन्तः		बलवन्तः
स्निग्ध ⇨	वर्ण	श्रुत
	स्वराः	वित्त
सन्धयश्च ⇨	स्थूल	विज्ञान
	दीर्घ	अपत्य
	वृत्त	सम्मानभाजश्च

7. Shukra Saara Pariksha:

Lakshana's of Shukra Saara:	It Indicates:
सौम्याः	
सौम्य प्रेक्षिणः(sight)? क्षीरपूर्णलोचना इव	
प्रहर्ष बहुलाः	ते स्त्री प्रियोपभोगा
स्निग्ध / शिखर दशनाः(tooth) (शिखरदशना इति ⇨ शोभनदशनाः)	बलवन्तः
वृत्त	सुख
सार	ऐश्वर्य
समसंहत	आरोग्य
	वित्त
प्रसन्न / वर्ण, स्वरा	सम्मान
स्निग्ध	आपत्य भाजश्च
भ्राजिष्णवो ? (kaanti vaan)	
महा स्फिचश्च - buttocks	

8. Satva Saara Pariksha:

Lakshana's of Satva Saara:	
स्मृतिमन्तो	समर विक्रान्त योधिन
भक्तिमन्तः	स्त्यक्त विषादाः
कृतज्ञाः - Gratitude	सुव्यवस्थित गति (स्वस्थिता इति न परस्थिताः)
प्राज्ञाः	गम्भीर बुद्धि चेष्टाः
शुचयो	कल्याणाभिनिवेशिनश्च (efforts)
महोत्साहा	तेषां स्वलक्षणैरेव गुणा व्याख्याताः
दक्षा	
धीराः	

Classification of Bala based on Saara;

Ati Bala	Madyama Bala	Alpa Bala
सर्वैः सारै रुप पुरुष- Present with lakshana's of all Saara's. Following Lakshanas are seen in them:	Madyama Saara – present with few of the Saara lakshans.	Asaara – present with lakshanas quite opposite to Sarva Saara Lakshana's
परमसुखयुक्ताः	Madyama	Alpa
क्लेशसहाः	Madyama	Alpa
सर्वारम्भेष्वात्मनि जातप्रत्ययाः	Madyama	Alpa
कल्याणाभिनिवेशिनः	Madyama	Alpa
स्थिर समाहित शरीराः	Madyama	Alpa
सुसमाहित गतयः	Madyama	Alpa
सानुनाद स्निग्ध गम्भीर महास्वराः	Madyama	Alpa
सुख	Madyama	Alpa
ऐश्वर्य	Madyama	Alpa
वित्त	Madyama	Alpa
उपभोग	Madyama	Alpa
सम्मानभाजो	Madyama	Alpa
मन्द जरसो	Madyama	Alpa
मन्द विकाराः	Madyama	Alpa
प्राय स्तुल्य गुण विस्तीर्णापत्या	Madyama	Alpa
चिरजीविनश्च	Madyama	Alpa

Samhanana Pariksha: Ch.Vi.8/116.

Synonymns: संहननं - संहतिः - संयोजन – एको sर्थः

Meaning: 'संहति इति निबिड सन्धान' (compactly joined)

Classification of Bala based on Samhana:

Balavanta	Madya Bala	Alpa Bala
सु संहत शरीराः पुरुषा बलवन्तः		
'सु संहतं शरीरम्' means	मध्यत्वात् संहननस्य मध्यबला	विपर्ययेणाल्पबलाः
1. सम सु विभक्त अस्थि - well oriented		
2. सु बद्ध सन्धि -well Knit		
3. सु निविष्ट मांस शोणितं - well bound		

The persons possessing the following qualities are not affected by Vyadhi bala of Vikaaras. Ch.Su.21/18
1. सम मांस प्रमाण
2. सम संहनन
3. दृढेन्द्रियो

Qualities of persons with **'सम मांस चयो'**: Ch.Su.21/19
1. क्षुत् पिपासा आतप सहः
2. शीत व्यायाम संसहः
3. सम पक्ता (Proper Digestion)
4. सम जरः (Proper Assimilation)

Pramana Pariksha: Ch.Vi.8/117

Pramana of Body parts as calculated by one's own Anguli's Breadth.

Pramaana of Avayava's in Anguli Pramana		Utseda	Vistaara	Ayama	Utseda / Parinaaha
		Height	Breadth	Length	Circumference
तत्र पादौ चत्वारि षट् चतुर्दशाङ्गुलानि	Paada	4	6	14	
जङ्घे त्वष्टादशाङ्गुले षोडशाङ्गुल परिक्षेपे च	Jangha			18	16
जानुनी चतुरङ्गुले षोडशाङ्गुल परिक्षेपे	Jaanu			4	16
त्रिंशदङ्गुल परिक्षेपा वष्टादशाङ्गुला वूरु	Uru			18	30
षडङ्गुल दीर्घौ वृषणा वष्टाङ्गुल परिणाहौ	Vrushana			6	8
शेफ: षडङ्गुल दीर्घं पञ्चाङ्गुल	Shepha			6	5

परिणाहं						
द्वादशाङ्गुलि परिणाहो भगः	Bhaga				12	
षोडशाङ्गुल विस्तारा कटी	Kati	16				
दशाङ्गुलं बस्ति शिरः	Basti Sira					10
दशाङ्गुल विस्तारं द्वादशाङ्गुल मुदरं	Udaram	10	12			
दशाङ्गुल विस्तीर्ण द्वादशाङ्गुलाया मे पार्श्वे	Paarshva	10	12			
द्वादशाङ्गुलं स्तनान्तरं	Sthana Antaram					12
द्व्यङ्गुलं स्तन पर्यन्तं	Sthana Paryantam					2
चतुर्विंशत्यङ्गुल विशालं द्वादशाङ्गुलोत्सेध मुरः	Uraha	12	24			
द्व्यङ्गुलं हृदयम्	Hrudayam					2

अष्टाङ्गुलौ स्कन्धौ	Skandou					8
षडङ्गुला वंसौ	Amsou					6
षोडशाङ्गुलौ प्रबाहू	Prabaahu (Rear Arm)			16		
पञ्चदशाङ्गुलौ प्रपाणी	Prapaani (Fore Arm)			15		
हस्तौ द्वादशाङ्गुलौ	Hastou			12		
कक्षा वष्टाङ्गुलौ	Kaksha			8		
त्रिकं द्वादशाङ्गुल उत्सेधम्	Trikam	12				
अष्टादशाङ्गुलो त्सेधं पृष्ठं	Prusta	18				
चतुरङ्गुलोत्सेधा द्वाविंशत्यङ्गुल परिणाहा शिरोधरा (Neck)	Shiro-Dharaa (Neck)	4			22	
द्वादशाङ्गुलोत्से धं चतुर्विंशत्यङ्गुल परिणाह माननं (Face)	Maanana (Face)	12			24	
पञ्चाङ्गुल मास्यं	Aasyam (Mouth)					5

चिबुक	Chibuka					4
ओष्ठ	Osta					4
कर्ण	Karna					4
अक्षि मध्य	Akshi Madya					4
नासिका	Nasika					4
ललाटं चतुरङ्गुलं	Lalatam (Fore Head)					4
षोडशाङ्गुलोत्सेधं द्वात्रिंशदङ्गुल परिणाहं शिरः	Shirah	16			32	

The Pramana of Complete Sharira is 84 Angulas (in length).

When the Breadth (calculated with out spread of arms) and Length of Sharira are equal. I; e. 84 Angulas. Such Proportions of Sharira is said of having '**Sama** Pramana' Sharira.
If the Proportions are alpa, said to have '**Hina** Pramana' Sharira.
If the Proportions are adhika, said to have '**Adhika** Pramana' Sharira.

The qualities like Ayu, bala, etc. are dependant on Sharira Pramana.

Sama Pramana	Hina Pramana	Adhika Pramana
Person with 'Sama Pramana' Sharira will attain the following qualities:	If the person is with 'Hina Pramana' Sharira will attain the Contrary qualities	If the person is with 'Adhika Pramana' Sharira will attain the Contrary qualities
आयु		
बलं		
ओजः		
सुख	Contrary qualities	
ऐश्वर्यं		
वित्तं		
इष्टा अपरे भावा (other Desires)		

Satmya Pariksha: Ch.Vi.8/118

Satmya: सात्म्यं नाम 'तद्यत् सातत्येन उपसेव्यमानम् उपशेते'

That which becomes useful / wholesome to body on continuous usage is said as Satmya.

Classification of Bala based on Satmya:

Balavanta Lakshana's	Madya Bala Lakshana's	Alpa Bala Lakshana's
घृत तैल क्षीर मांसरस सात्म्याः	व्यामिश्र सात्म्यास्तु	रूक्ष सात्म्याः
सर्व रस सात्म्याश्च	Mixed	एक रस सात्म्याश्च (पञ्चरसा असात्म्यत्वेनापथ्या)
क्लेश सहा	Mixed	अल्प क्लेश सहा
चिर जीविनश्च	Mixed	अल्पायुषो
Bahu Sadhana (Beshaja)	Mixed	ऽल्प साधनाश्च (अल्पभेषजाः)

Satva Pariksha: Ch.Vi.8/119.

'सत्त्वमुच्यते मनः'

तत् शरीरस्य तन्त्रकम् आत्म संयोगात् | (तन्त्रकमिति प्रेरक धारकं च)

Satva is the Preraka & Dhaaraka of Sharira, due to its samyoga with Atma.

Satvam is of 3 types based on its Bala:	Also Purusha are of 3 types based on Satva Bala
प्रवरं	प्रवर सत्त्व पुरुष
मध्यम्	मध्य सत्त्व पुरुष
अवरं	अवर सत्त्व पुरुष

Classification of Bala based on Satva:

प्रवर सत्त्वाः	मध्य सत्त्वाः	हीन सत्त्वाः		
1. Possessed with the **lakshana's** of **Satva Saara**. 2. Though with alpa sharira & inspite of being affected by strong, painful nija or agantu vyadhi's, they look as if painless, due to their Satva guna visesha.	1. They themselves make their support (console / comfort / condition) by taking others point of view in to their account or else depends on support of others.	1. They don't intend in making support of their own or from other's satva bala. 2. Though with maha sharira, they seem incapable of bearing even slight pains or weak ailments. 3.		

when they face	Hear the Stories of	At the sight of
भय	रौद्र	पशु पुरुष
शोक	भैरव	मांस
लोभ	द्विष्ट	शोणितानि
मोह	बीभत्स	
माना:	विकृत	

They attain:

Any of the following				
विषाद	मूर्च्छ	भ्रम	or	मरणम्
वैवर्ण्य	उन्माद	प्रपतनानाम्		

Ahara Shakti Pariksha: Ch.Vi.8/120.

Ahara Shakti is known from:

1. Abyavaharana Shakti – bhojana Shakti / Capacity to Consume.

2. Jarana Shakti – Pachana Shakti / Capacity to Digest.

'जरणशक्त्या च इति वचनादि यो बहु भुङ्क्ते परिणमयति'
'Ahara' provides both:

1. Bala &
2. Ayu

or else can say, Bala & Ayu are dependent on Ahara.

Vyayama Shakti Pariksha: Ch.Vi.8/121

Vyayama Shakti is known from 'Karma Shakti.'

Based on 'Karma Shakti,' 'Bala traividya' is inferred.

Here 'Karma' means bhaara vahana, etc.

Vayaha Pariksha: Ch.Vi.8/122

Vayaha:

'वयस्तश्चेति काल प्रमाण विशेषापेक्षिणी हि शरीरावस्था वयो ऽभिधीयते.'

The Sharia avastha, which is based on Kaala Paramana Visesha is Vayah. Upon Sthula Bheda, Vayaha is of 3 kinds:

बालं		मध्यं	जीर्ण
अपरि पक्व धातु	विवर्धमान धातु गुणं	समत्वागत	अतः परं क्रमेण
अजात व्यञ्जनं	प्रायेण अनवस्थित सत्त्वं	बल	हीय मान धात्विन्द्रिय बल
सुकुमारं		वीर्य	वीर्य
अक्लेशसहं	आत्रिंशद्वर्ष	पौरुष	पौरुष
असम्पूर्ण बलं		पराक्रम	पराक्रम
श्लेष्म धातु प्राय	Till 30 years	ग्रहण	ग्रहण
आषोडश वर्ष		धारण	धारण
		स्मरण	स्मरण
		वचन	वचन
		विज्ञान	विज्ञानं
Till 16 years		सर्व धातु गुणं	भ्रश्यमान धातुगुणं
		बल स्थित	वायु धातु प्रायं
		अवस्थित सत्त्व	आवर्षशतम् - Till 100 years
		अविशीर्यमाण धातुगुणं	
		पित्त धातु प्रायं	
		आषष्टि वर्ष - Till 60 years	

During the present period, the Ayu Pramana is 100 years. Of course, there are people who live for a longer or shorter period than this. Their vayaha should be classified by knowing the Ayu Pramana with the help of

1. Prakrti etc. bala visesha, excluding Vikruti and
2. Lakshana's of Ayu.

Ayu Pramana is determined by	
1. Prakruti etc. examination: (except Vikruti)	2. Lakshana's of Ayu:
Bala is classified into 3 varities: Pravara, Avara, Madyama.	Classified into Pravara, Avara, Madyama.

On basis of Ayu Pramana I; e. Pravara, Avara, Madyama. Vayah can be divided in to 3 kinds: Pravara, Avara, Madyama.

Pravara Vayaha:

Persons are with Ayu Pramana is > 100 years.
Ex: - If the person has a Ayu pramana of 120 years.

Bala: Vayaha	Madya: Vayaha	Vrudda: Vayaha
Till 36 years	Till 72 years	Remaining period

Madyama Vayaha:

Persons are with Ayu Pramana is < 100 years.
Ex: - If the person has a Ayu pramana of 80 years

Bala: Vayaha	Madya: Vayaha	Vrudda: Vayaha
Till 25 years	Till 50 years	Remaining period

Avara Vayaha:

They live till 20 years only and wont reach to Madya avastha of vayah.

From the above said 10 Factors,

'**Deha bala**' visesha can be calculated from 'Prakruti etc. (except Vikruti)':

Prakruti etc. (except Vikruti): ⊏⟩		Deha Bala Visesha Vibhajana:
Prakruti :	Satva	1. Pravara Bala
Saara :	Ahaara Shakti	2. Madya Bala
Samhanana	Vyayama Shakti	3. Avara Bala
Pramana	Vayah	
Satmya		

Anumaana of '**Trividha Dosha Bala**' can be had from '**Trividha Vikruti Bala.**'

Trividha Vikruti Bala: ⊏⟩	Trividha Dosha Bala
1. Pravara Vikruti Bala	1. Pravara Dosha Bala
2. Madya Vikruti Bala	2. Madya Dosha Bala
3. Avara Vikruti Bala	3. Avara Dosha Bala

Depending on the '**Trividha Dosha Bala**,' '**Trividha Bhaishajya**' is administered.

Trividha Dosha Bala ⊏⟩	Trividha Bhaishajya
1. Pravara Dosha Bala	1. Tikshna Bhaishajya
2. Madya Dosha Bala	2. Madya Bhaishajya
3. Avara Dosha Bala	3. Mridu Bhaishajya

Shat Kriya Kaala: Su.Su.21/18.

Kriya Kaala:

The 'Kaala' to perform 'Kriya' is 'Kriya Kaala.' i; e. the proper Time for Chikitsa Karma.

There are 6 Specific Time Period's for Medical Intervention with respect to Disease progression.

1. Sanchaya: Su.Su.21/18.

प्रथमः क्रियाकालः आद्यः कर्मावसरः

It is the 1st Time period for Chiktsa Karma (Medical intervention).

संहतीरूपा वृद्धिश्चयः

The Samhata Rupa Vruddi is Chaya I, e. Dosha Vruddi occurs due to their accumulation.

Due to the Dosha Sanchaya Hetu's, Dosha's get Sanchaya in 'Dosha Sthana's, producing Lakshana's as given below.

Dosha Sanchaya Lakshana's :

Sanchaya:	Vata	Pitta	Kapha
Lakshana's:	Stabdha	Peeta Avabaasata	Gowravam
	Poorna Kostata	Manda Ushmata	Alasyam
General Lakshana:	Chaya Kaarana Vidwesha		

| | 2. Prakopa | Su.Su.21/27. |

द्वितीयः क्रियाकाल इति द्वितीयश्चिकित्सावसरः

It is the 2nd Time period for Chiktsa Karma (Medical intervention).

विलयनरूपा वृद्धिः प्रकोपः

The Vilayana Rupa Vruddi is Prakopa I, e. Dosha Vruddi occurs due their melting State.

Due to the Dosha Prakopaka Hetu's, Dosha's get Prakopa in 'Dosha Sthana's due to Vilayana, & produce Lakshana's as given below.

Dosha Prakopa Lakshana's:

Prakopa:	Vata	Pitta	Kapha
Lakshana's:	Kosta Toda	Amla Udgaara	Anna Dwesha
	Kosta Samcharana (Pari- Bhramana)	Pipaasa (Thirst) Paridaaha (Sarvato Daaha)	Hrudaya utkleda (Hrillasa) (Nausea)

| | 3. Prasara: | Su.Su.21/28. |

तृतीयः क्रियाकालः

It is the 3rd Time period for Chiktsa Karma (Medical intervention).

The dosha's which reached the state of Prakopa, turns into Prasara due to their further Slight Vitiation (hetu balena udrikta dosha's).

Dosha Prasara occurs like as in case of mixture of yeast, water and flour there is excitation and overflowing due to mutual interaction, the same takes place in case of vata etc. in combination of various causative factors.

Difference between Prakopa & Prasara:

स्त्यानस्य सर्पिषः क्वाथ्यमानस्य प्रथमं सञ्चलनमात्रमेव **प्रकोपः**, तस्यैव चातिक्वाथ्यमानस्य फेनमण्डलेनोत्सर्पता देशान्तरसरणमिव **प्रसरः**|

when solid ghee is heated, at first there is only some movement - this is **prakopa** and when it overflows and begins to spread here and there with foamy incircling – it is **prasara**.

If the Dosha's are not aggravated potently, they stay hidden in channels for a while (Leena) and as time goes on and if no measures are taken to treat then they get aggravated by their causative factors leading to Dosha Prasara.

The kaarana for the Prasarana is Gati of Vayu. Vayu is Rajo predominant & is the initiator of all Bhava's (Padartha's).

As a large accumulation of water further excessively increased breaks the barrier and mixes with other pool of water & run in all directions. So also Doshas spread sometimes alone or in combinations of two or all or with Rakta in 15 ways.

Vata	Vata Pitta	Vata-Pitta-Kapha
Pitta	Vata Kapha	Vata-Pitta-Rakta
Kapha	Vata Rakta	Vata-Kapha-Rakta
Rakta	Pitta Kapha	Pitta-Kapha-Rakta
	Pitta Rakta	
	Kapha Rakata	Vata-Pitta-Kapha-Rakta

क्रिया विभागः (Classification of Dosha Chikitsa): Su.Su.21/31

'प्रसरेण अन्य दोष स्थान गतस्य दोषस्य स्थानिवत् प्रतीकार'

'दोषस्थान गतं दोषं स्थानिवत् समुपाचरेत्'

Vata Dosha on reaching Pitta Sthana should be tackled by Pitta Chikitsa,

Pitta Dosha on reaching Kapha Sthana should be tackled by Kapha Chikitsa and

Kapha Dosha on reaching Vata Sthana should be tackled by Vata Chikitsa.

Ex:-

Prasarita Dosha	Prasarita Sthana	Sthanivat Chikitsa = Sthanika Dosha Chikitsa
Vata	Pitta Sthana	Pitta Doshavat Chikitsa
Vata	Kapha Sthana	Kapha Doshavat Chikitsa
Pitta	Vata Sthana	Vata Doshavat Chikitsa
Pitta	Kapha Sthana	Kapha Doshavat Chikitsa
Kapha	Vata Sthana	Vata Doshavat Chikitsa
Kapha	Pitta Sthana	Pitta Doshavat Chikitsa

Though there are 15 types of Prasara yet Chikitsa is limited to 3 Dosha's only.

Dosha Prasara Lakshana's:

	Vata	Pitta	Kapha
Lakshana's:	Vayu Vimarga Gamana (प्रकृतवायुमार्गादन्यो विमार्गः) Atopa (आटोपो रुजापूर्वक उदरक्षोभः)	Osha (ओष एकदेशिको दाहः) Chosha (चोषः चूष्यत इव वेदनाविशेषः) Paridaaha (Sarvato Daaha) Dhumaayanam	Arochaka Avipaka AngaSaada Chardhi

तत्र प्रसरं यावद्दोषाणामेव हेतुलिङ्गचिकित्सा, तदनन्तरं व्याधेरिति

Till this state of Prasara, Chikitsa is given only for Hetu and Linga of dosas and the state thereafter is the disease & its treatment.

4. Sthana Samshrayam: Su.Su.21/33.
चतुर्थः क्रियाकाल इति चतुर्थश्चिकित्सावसरः|

It is 4th Time period for Chiktsa Karma (Medical intervention).

प्रसृतानां पुनर्दोषाणां स्रोतोवैगुण्याद्यत्र सङ्गः स स्थानसंश्रयः

The Doshas which are in Prasara avsatha gets Sangha in the Srotas at a place which became vaigunya (abnormal). Such a Sanga is said as 'Sthana Samshraya.'

तत्र स्रोतो वैगुण्याद्यत्र सक्ता यान् यान् रोगान् कुर्विन्ति तांस्तान् निर्देष्टुमाह

The Rogas that occur due to sanga of the Doshas in the respective Srotases are said below:

or

एवं प्रकुपितातांस्ताऱ् शरीरप्रदेशानागम्य तांस्तान् व्याधीन् जनयन्ति |

The prakupita doshas reach Sharira Pradesha's and cause Diseases of respective Pradesha are as follows.

In उदर	बस्तिगताः	मेढ्रगता	गुदगता	वृषणगता	ऊर्ध्वजत्रुगता
गुल्म	प्रमेहा	निरुद्धप्रकशो	भगन्दर	वृद्धीः	ऊर्ध्वजान्
विद्रधि	अश्मरी	उपदंश	अर्शः		
उदर	मूत्राघात	शूकदोष	Etc.		
अग्निसङ्ग	मूत्रदोष	Etc.			
आनाह	Etc.				
विसूचिका					
अतिसार					
प्रवाहिका					
विलम्बिका					
Etc.					

त्वङ्मंसशोणितस्थाः	मेदोगता	अस्थिगता	पादगताः	सर्वाङ्ग गता
क्षुद्ररोगान्	ग्रन्थि	विद्रधि	श्लीपद	ज्वर
कुष्ठानि	अपचि	अनुशयी (Boil)	वातशोणित	सर्वाङ्ग रोग
विसर्पाश्च	अर्बुद	Etc.	वातकण्टक	प्रमेह
	गलगण्डा		Etc.	पाण्डुरोग
Here Twak = Rasa Dathu	अलजी			शोष
	Etc.			Etc.

When the Doshas are established in this way, Purvarupa which is disease specific gets appeared. Purvarupa avastha denotes the 4th Kriya kaala. Or 4nd Time period for Chiktsa Karma (Medical intervention).

सूक्ष्मत्वात् स्थानसंश्रयस्य न पृथगुक्तं लक्षणं, न अपि क्रियाकाल

Due to sukshmatva stage of Sthana Samshraya, Lakshana's & Treatment are not said separately I, e. both are said while describing the disease.

चिकित्सा चात्र दोषस्य दूष्यस्य चेत्युभयाश्रिता

In this Time Period, the Chikitsa is Ubhaya Ashrita I, e. on Dosha's & Dushya's.

5. Vyakti: Su.Su.21/34.

पञ्चमः क्रियाकालः

It is 5th Time period for Chiktsa Karma (Medical intervention).

व्याधेः प्रव्यक्तं रूपं व्यक्तिः

The 'Rupa PraVyakta' of Vyadhi is said as 'Vyakti.'

Here, the 'Vyadhi Darshana' occurs by 'PraVyakta Lakshana's.

'PraVyakta Lakshana' means 'Vyadhi Jati Lakshana'.

Examples:-
1. 'Dosha Samghatha with Twak, Mamsa sthana's' in causing Shopha, Arbuda,
Granthi, Vidradi, Visarpa etc.
2. 'Santapa' Lakshana in Jwara.
3. 'Sarana' Lakshana in Atisara.
4. 'Purana' Lakshana in Udara. Etc.

अत्र व्याधेः प्रत्यनीकैव चिकित्सा

In this Time period, Chikitsa is Pratyanika to the Vyadhi. I; e. treatment contrary to disease is given.

6. Bhedam   Su.Su.21/35.

षष्ठः क्रियाकालः

It is 6th Time period for Chiktsa Karma (Medical intervention).

After the Vyakti avstha, Shopha, Arbuda, Granthi, Vidradi, Visarpa etc. undergo avadeerna (burst / torn) and become Vrana (ulcers).

In case of Jwara, Atisara etc. they attain 'Dheerga Kaala Anubandha' (chronicity).

Such Specific Nature of turning into Avadeerana / Dheergha kaala Anubandha is the Bhedha (Specification).

If chikitsa is not adopted in these 6 Kriya Kaala's they turn into Asadya.

The person with knowledge regarding 'Shat Kriya Kaala's' of Dosha's is considered as 'Bhishak.'

The vitiated doshas if treated in 'Sanchaya' avastha donot move into further avastha's. On moving into further avastha's they become 'Balavattara.'
I; e.
- o 'Pratikaara Alpatva' is only needed in Primary Stages of 'Kriya kaala.'
- o 'Pratikaara Bahulya' is needed in Later Stages of 'Kriya Kaala.'

Dosha Prakopa & Chikitsa:

The Dosha Kupitha occurs with

    a. All of the Bhava's (Factors)
    b. 3 of the Bhava's
    c. 2 of the Bhava's
    d. 1 of the Bhava.

Here the word ' Bhava' which are the Vyadhi Hetu's: they can be any of the following:

Vyadhi hetu's (Bhava's)			
A	**B**	**C**	**D**
Ahara	Rasa	Dravya	Dosha Bhaaga's acc. to others
Vihara	Guna	Guna	Ruksha. Lahu, Vishada, Vishtambha etc. of Vata.
Desha	Veerya	Karma	Tikshna, Drava, puti, nila, peeta etc of Pitta.
Kaala	Vipaka	As per Bhattar Harishhandra, commentator of Charaka	Sita, Guru, Picchila, Snigdha etc. of Kapha.

- The Bhaagaa's by which the doshas get vitiated, the chikitsa should be adopting the opposite bhaagaa's with respect to those vitiated.

Example:

1.

Dosha affected	Dosha Bhaagaas affeccted	Chikitsa with the Bhaaga
Vata	1 Bhaagaa	
	Ruksha	Snigdha

2.

Dosha affected	Dosha Bhaagaas affeccted	Chikitsa with the Bhaagas
Vata	2 Bhaagaas	
	Ruksha	Snigdha
	Sita	Ushna

Similarly treated if affeccted by all the Bhavas also.

In the Samsarga state of Dosha':

If a Dosha is said to be krudda with respect to other, if it is vitiated with 'All the Bhava's', such a dosha is said as **Anubandhya** Dosha / **Pradhana**/ **Primary** Dosha.

The other left over Dosha is said as **Anubandha** Dosha / **Apradhana**/ **Secondary** Dosha, which may be vitiated with '3/2/1 bhavas.'

Such a Secondary Dosha moves along with (Anu Dhaavathi) Primary dosha. Hence Chikitsa of primary Dosha also pacifies the Secondary Dosha.

The Chikitsa of the Primary Dosha is adopted in such a way so that it should not be like Virodha to the Secondary Doshas I, e. This should not vitiate the secondary Doshas.
Two types of Samsarga is possible:

1. Prakriti Sama Samaveta Samsarga
2. Vikriti Vishama Samaveta Samsarga
If,

Dosha involveed	Showing Svabhava Sadrishsa
Vata	Shoshanatmaka
Pitta	Shoshanatmaka

This is Prakriti Sama Samaveta Samsarga of doshas.

If,

Dosha involveed	Showing Svabhava Viparita
Pitta	Ushnam
Kapha	Shitam

This is Vikriti Vishama Samaveta Samsarga of doshas.

This can be applied in case of Sannipata Doshas too.

Nidaana Panchaka in Roga Pariksha:

हेतुलिङ्गज्ञानपूर्विका हि चिकित्सा साध्वी भवति|

ch.ni.1/1 commentary.

Chikitsa becomes possible after attaining gnana of Hetu & Linga.

The vyadhi Gnana is attained by these 5 upaayaas also said as Nidana Panchaka's

1. Nidaana
2. Purvarupa
3. Linga
4. Upashaya
5. Samprapti

1. Nidana:

Nidaana is the Kaarana.It Provides information regarding:-

1. Vyaadhi Janakam	2. Vyaadhi Bhodhakam ('व्याधि ज्ञान जनकं')
The Nidaanam in respect to Vyaadhi janaka is the Hetu.	Vyaadhi Bhodaka occurs from kaaranas like "Nidaana,Purvarupa, Rupa, Upashaya, Samprapti."

Synonymns:

Hetu: "हेतुरकृतकत्वात्" (वि.अ.८/31)

Nimitta:

Ayatanam: "दशैवायतनानि स्युः" (सू.अ.२९/3)

Karthaa:

Kaaranam:

Pratyaya: "कर्ता, मन्ता, वेदिता, बोद्धा" (शा.अ.४) इत्यादौ, प्रत्ययस्य लडादौ

Samutthaanam: उत्थानस्य उद्गमनादौ

Nidaanam:

योनि

मूल

मुख

प्रकृत्यादयो

3 kinds of **Nidaana** are Possible for causation of a Vyaadhi.

1. असात्म्येन्द्रियार्थसंयोगः

2. प्रज्ञापराधः

3. परिणाम

These are the only 3 possibilties for causation of a Vyaadhi and not more other. Among these, mula Kaarana is Asatmya indriyaartha samyoga.

Sannikrista Kaarna & Viprakrista Kaarna

कारणं च व्याधीनां सन्निकृष्टं वातादि,

विप्रकृष्टं चार्थानामयोगादि;

पुनर्विप्रकृष्टं कारणं रक्तपित्तस्य ज्वरसन्ताप इत्यादि;

पुनश्च व्याधीनां सामान्येन विप्रकृष्टं कारणमुक्तं

यथा- "प्रागपि चाधर्मादृते न रोगोत्पत्तिरभूत्" (वि.अ.३) इत्यादि;

2. Purvarupa:

पूर्वरूपं प्रागुत्पत्ति लक्षणं व्याधेः ||८||

The lakshana seen before the vyadhi Utpatti is said as **Purvarupa**.

"स्थान संश्रयिणः क्रुद्धा भावि व्याधि प्रबोधकम्| लिङ्गं कुर्वन्ति यद्दोषाः पूर्वरूपं तदुच्यते" इति|

Prakupita doshas in the state of 'Sthaana Samshraya' causes "Bhaavi Vyaadhi Prabhodakam" by producing Lingam respective to the doshas, which is said as **Purvarupa**.

By seeing condition of Clouds, Rain can be Anumiyate (inferred) & by seeing Udayam of rohini Nakshatra, Krittika Udaya is also inferred. Similarly a Disease can be Inferred from its Purvarupa's.

तच्च पूर्वरूपं द्विविधम्-

Samanya Purvarupa	Vishista Purvarupa
दोष दूष्य सम्मूर्च्छन अवस्था जनितं, भावि ज्वरादि व्याधि मात्रं प्रतीयते, नतु वातादि जनितत्वादि विशेष:	भावि व्याधि लिङ्गानाम अव्यक्तत्वम् or भावि व्याधि अव्यक्त रूपं
Purvarupas other than Avyakta Lingam	अव्यक्तं लक्षणं - मल्पत्वाद्व्याधीनां - अल्पत्वेन - अणुत्वात् - न अत्यभिव्यक्तम् - अस्फुटत्वम् - (found in Alpa, not clear.).
The Purvarupa found in relation to Dosha Dushya Sammurchana Avastha provide us to know about the Vyadhi only. But not Dosha visesha.	It gives an idea about the dosa visesha in Vyadhi.
	In Jwara, विशेषात्तु जृम्भास्त्यर्थं समीरणात्। पित्तान्नयनयोर्दाहः कफान्नान्नाभिनन्दनम्"

पूर्वरूपत्रैविध्यं दर्शितं- अरुणदत्तेन तु (वाग्भटव्याख्यायां)

Purva rupa is of 3 types:

1. शारीरं,

2. मानसं,

3. शारीरमानसं च।

There are niyata purvarupas in the purvarupa stage of vyaadhi.

In the purvarupa avastha only vyadhi gnana occurs.

3. Lingam

प्रादुर्भूत लक्षणं पुनर्लिङ्गम्।

The produced lakshana's are said as **Lingam**.

तथा वातादयाम पक्वादि विशेषण विशिष्टं व्याधिं निदानोपशय सम्प्राप्ति व्यतिरिक्तं यद्बोधयति, तल्लिङ्गम्।

The lakshanas that says about a vyaadhi which are due to Vaataadi, pakvaadi viseshana visistam and not including lakshanas of Nidaana –Upashaya – samprapti. Such Lakshanas are said to be Lingam.

The synonymns are:

Lingam	Chihnam	Rupam
Akruti	Samsthaanam	
Lakshanam	Vyanjanam	

अनेन च व्याधि प्रतिनियतं लिङ्गं यथा- vyadhi prati niyata Lingam are said as:

1. ज्वरस्य सन्तापः,
2. तथा अतिसरणम अतीसारस्य इत्यादि गृह्यते;
3. तथा वातादिकृतं च वातादि ज्वरस्य - -> विषमारम्भ विसर्गित्वादि गृह्यते;
4. तथा आम, पक्व, जीर्ण ज्वर लक्षणादीनि - - >विशिष्ट व्याधि बोधकानि गृह्यन्ते;
5. तथा उपद्रवा,श्चासाध्यतादय, अवस्थ - - >आपन्न व्याधि बोधकत्वेन लक्षणान्येव।
6. रिष्टं तु मरणस्य पूर्वरूपमेव।

In Rupa avastha, dosha visesha gnana of vyadhi occurs.

4. Upashaya:

उपशयस्तु चिकित्सा,

That which establishes Sukhaanubandha when taken in form of Oushadha, Ahaara & Vihaara with respect to stages of a Disease.

They are as:

1. Hetu Viparita Upashaya
2. Vyadhi Viparita Upashaya
3. Hetu & Vyadhi Viparita Upashaya
4. Hetu Viparita Arthakaari Upashaya
5. Vyadhi Viparita Arthakaari Upashaya
6. Hetu & Vyadhi Viparita Arthakaari Upashaya

Viparita Arthakari' means:-

अत्र च विपरीतार्थकारि तदेवोच्यते यदविपरीत तया ऽऽपाततः प्रतीयमानं विपरीतस्यार्थं प्रशम लक्षणं करोति|

Viparita Arthakaari is that which is not viparita (opposite in action) but for a moment it gives result of Viparita Artham which is shown in form of prashama Lakshana.

Upashaya provides Gyana upaaya of both

1. The Vyadhi &
2. The Gooda Lingaas.

The Gooda lingas in a Vyaadhi are to be examined with help of Upashaya & Anupashaya.

Ex:-
The Shotha, if it gets treated by using Sneha-Ushna-Mardana. Such a Shotha can be known or diagnosed to be vaatika type of Shotha.

Upashaya Bhedas are as:

	Upashaya	Oushada	Ahara	Vihaara
1.	Hetu viparita	Ushna oushada prayoga in vaata jwara	Mamsa rasa with anna in shrama janita vaata jwara	Awaken in night for the vrudda kapha due to day sleep
2.	Vyadhi viparita	Sirisha twak in visha vikaras, shunti in atisaara	Stambhaka dravya in atisaara (masoora), barley in prameha	Pravahana in udavarta and balidaana, praayaschitta etc.
3.	Hetu vyadhi viparita	Dashamoola quath in vataja shota	Takra in vata kapha grahani, peya prayoga in vaata jwara	Ratri jaagarana in diva swaapa janita tandraa
4.	Hetu viparita artha kaaraka	Pitta vardaka upanaaha in pittaja vrana shota	Vidaahi anna etc. in pachyamaana vrana shota	Bhaya kaaraka prayoga in vaataja unmaada
5.	Vyadhi viparita artha kaaraka	Vamana kaaraka madaphala prayoga in chardi roga	Virechanaartha dugdha prayoga in pittaja atisaara	Pravaahana (vamana) prayoga in chardi roga
6.	Hetu vyadhi viparita artha kaaraka	Ushna aguru etc. lepa on agni dagdha	Punah Madhya paana in adhika madhyapaana janita madaatyaya	Swimming in river in vyaayaama janita vaata vikruti

Anupashaya also useful for Pariksha of Vyaadhi, it is as follows:

The One which is Viparita to upashaya is Anupashaya, also it is memorised as Asatmya.

Such Anupashaya can be considered under Nidaana only. So Anupashya is not said separately.

More over hetu sevana causes Anupashaya.

5. Samprapti:-

"यथा दुष्टेन दोषेण यथा चानु विसर्पता|
निर्वृत्ति रामयस्यासौ सम्प्राप्ति र्जाति रागति: [२] " (वा. नि.अ.१)

सम्प्राप्ति र्जाति रागति रित्यनर्थान्तरं व्याधे:

The dusta doshas with its Anu-Visarpana causes Aamaya. Such a process is called as Samprapti or jaati or Agati.

Though after samprapti only occurrence of Linga occurs, yet due to its alpa Prayojana in the Vyadhi nirupana(gnana) it is said at last as 'Samprapti etc.'

The description of an Artha (vishaya/topic) if said by using the words 'Samprapti, Agati, Jaati', it denotes the 'Samprapti' of the Vyadhi.

Jaati:-

जाति: जन्म
Jaati means Janma (starting point).

व्याधि जनक दोष व्यापार विशेष युक्तं व्याधि जन्मेह सम्प्राप्ति:
The association of vyaadhi janaka visesha dosha vyaapaara causes vyadhi janma, is the 'Samprapti'.

Agati:-

आगतिर्हि उत्पादकारणस्य व्याधि जनन पर्यन्तं गमनम्|

The gamanam from Utpaadaka kaarana till the Vyaadhi janana is the 'Agati'.

Such Samprapti gives the Bhodha (understanding) of Vyadhi Visesham.

Ex: - यथा ज्वरे-

'स यदा प्रकुपितः प्रविश्यामाशयम्' इत्यारभ्य 'तदा ज्वरमभिनिर्वर्तयति'

इत्यन्तेन या सम्प्राप्तिरुच्यते, तया

ज्वरस्यामाशयदूषकत्वाग्न्युपघातकत्वरसदूषकत्वादयो धर्माः प्रतीयन्ते|

Jwara Samprapti is said as to start from 'स यदा प्रकुपितः

प्रविश्यामाशयम्' till 'तदा ज्वरमभिनिर्वर्तयति'.

By saying so 'Amaashaya Dushakatva, Agni Upaghaatakatva, Rasa pradushakatva etc. Dharma's of Jwara can understood.

ततश्च कारणधर्माणां निदानग्रहणेनैव ग्रहणं भवतीति; यतः,

कारणधर्मोऽप्ययं व्याधिजनकदोषव्यापाररूपः

'Kaarana Dharma's' are understood just by Understanding 'Nidaana.' Hence, 'Kaarana Dharma' itself is the 'Dosha Vyaapaara rupam' with respect to Vyadhi janaka.

Samprapti Bhedha's:-

सा सङ्ख्या प्राधान्य विधि विकल्प बल काल विशेषै र्भिद्यते

The Samprapti is divided based on its visesha's like Saamkhya, Praadhaanya, Vidhi, Vikalpa, Bala, Kaala.

Samprapti is different for different vyaadhi's & Vyakti's.

The samprapti gets divided by Samkhya etc. vyadhi's also gets divided by samkhya etc.

Samkhya Samprapti:-

सङ्ख्या तावद्यथा- अष्टौ ज्वराः, पञ्च गुल्माः, सप्तकुष्ठान्येवमादिः|१२|

8 types of Jwara, 5 types of Gulma, 7 types of Kusta etc.

After saying 8 types of jwara, 2 types of Rakta Pitta is not said in an order because 2 types of Rakta Pitta is said based on Vidhi Bhedha not by Saamkhya Bhedha.

Pradhanya Samprapti:-

Praadhaanya tells about the 'Tara', 'Tama' of Doshas. Regarding vruddi of doshas those 2 shabdha's are used.

'Tara'	'Tama'
'Tara' is based on 2 doshas,	'Tama' is based on 3 doshas.
'Tara' is based on vruddi among the 2 doshas.	'Tama' is based on vruddi among the 3 doshas.
In dwi doshaja vikaaras, in saying about the praadhanyata of one dosha among the two, 'Tara' word is used.	In Tri doshaja vikaaras, in saying about the praadhnyata of one dosha among the three, 'Tama' word is used.

Vidhi Samprapti:-

विधि रिति विधि कृत इत्यर्थः|

Based on which, the division is done. Such basis is the 'vidhi'.

विधिश्च प्रकारो भेद इत्यर्थः|

The meaning of 'Vidhi' is Prakaara & Bhedha.

	Kinds of Vyadhi		
	2	**3**	**4**
Based on	Nija	Vataja	Sadya
	Agantu	Pittaja	Asadya
		Kaphaja	Mridhu
			Daaruna

Based on	Sadya	Asadya
Mridhu	Mridu Sadya = Sukha Sadya	Mridu Asadya = Yapya
Daaruna	Daaruna Sadya = Krichra Sadya	Daaruna Asadya = Pratyakyeya

Vikalpa Samprapti:-

समवेतानां [१] पुनर्दोषाणामंशांश बल विकल्पो विकल्पो sस्मिन्नर्थे|१२|

The word smavetha denotes Sarva doshas in a vyadhi. Singly, dually & combined form of doshas are considered.

Bala pertaining to each Amsha of Dosha is **Amsha-Amsha Bala** of Dosha.

Utkarsha, Apkarsha rupa vikalpa of Amsha-Amsha Bala of the Dosha's is **Amsha-Amsha Bala Vikalpa**.

The combined doshas in a vyaadhi & their amshaamsha Bala Vikalpa is **Vikalpa Samprapthi**.

Amshama Dosha Vikalpa is said as: In the Vata prakopa, it may be due to Sita Amsha or some times due to Laghu Amsha or Ruksha Amsha or sometimes Laghu-Ruksha Amsha, etc.	The Amsha Amsha Bala Vikalpa of the Dosha's is produced by the gunas of Dosha's due to difference in the Hetu.
Similarly Pitta & Kapha Amsha-Amsha Vikalpa Udaharana can be taken.	

Bala Kaala Samprapti:

The time (Kaala) at which dosha's are in Bala Avastha or disesase is in Bala Avastha. Such a period is **bala Kaala.**

Ex: - Vasanta, Purvahna etc. Bala kaala visehsa's.

Based on the following:-	Vyaadhi or Dosa - Bala kaala Depends:-
Rithu, Ahoratra, Ahaara Kaala. **Ex:-**	Vidhi Viniyata (Vinischaya) of Vyaadhi or 'Bala-Kaala-Visesha,' of Vyadhi.
Vi-Niyata of Rithu	Sleshma jwara in Vasantha Rithu kaala.
Vi-Niyata of Ahoratra	Sleshma jwara in Purvahna kaala and Pradosha Kaala.
Vi-Niyata of Ahaara	Sleshma jwara in Bhukta Maatra Kaala.

Importance of Nidana Panchaka's in Roga Pariksha:

तस्माद्व्याधीन् भिषगनुपहत सत्त्व बुद्धि हेंत्वादिभि र्भावै र्यथा

वदनुबुद्ध्येत   Ch.Ni.1/13.

A Bhishak should understand the vyaadhi'as it is' with Anupahata Satva,Buddhi, Hetvaadi Bhaava's.

यस्मादिमे निदानादय उक्तेन न्यायेन व्याधिपरीक्षायामुपयुक्ताः

तस्माद्व्याधीन् भिषग् हेत्वादिभिः परीक्षेतेति योजना

The said nidaanaadi are upayukta in vyaadhi pariksha. Hence a bhishak should do yojana of hetvaadi in the pariksha of vyadhi.

तत्र यो निदानं विस्मृतवान्, तस्य पूर्वरूपादिभिर्व्याधिः परीक्ष्यते

तथा यत्र च पूर्वरूपादयो विस्मृताः सन्दिग्धा वा, तत्रोपशयेन परीक्षा भवति

If at all one forgets Nidaana, then the vyadhi pariksha is done using purvarupa's, also if forgets or in confused state about the purvarupa's, then vyadhi parisha is done using Upashaya.

Ashta Sthana Rogi Pariksha

(Yogaratnakara.Purva Khanda - रोगिनामष्ट स्थान निरीक्षणम्)

रोगाक्रान्त शरीरस्य स्थानानि अष्टौ निरीक्षयेत् |

नाडीं मूत्रं मलं जिह्वां शब्दं स्पर्शं दृक् आकृती ||१||

The Sharira affected with Roga should be examined at 8 sthanas. They are:

1. Naadi
2. Mutra
3. Mala
4. Jihva
5. Shabdha
6. Sparsha
7. Drik
8. Akruti

In the examination of any diesase, these 8 are to be examined at first before initiating the Chikitsa.

Keeping in view about Knowledge of Desha, Kaala, Roga – Bala & Abala, then the vaidya should start Chikitsa, which brings him Yashas & Keerthi.

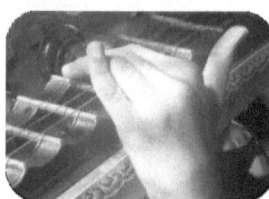

1. Naadi Pariksha:

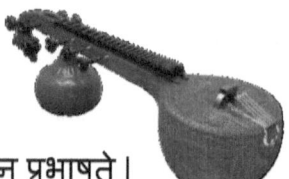

यथा वीणागता तन्त्री सर्वान् रागान् प्रभाषते |

तथा हस्तगता नादी सर्वान् रागान् प्रकाशयेत् ||३||

Just as the Tantra's in a **Veena** can produce all the Raaga's, in same way Hastagata Naadi too can illustrate all types of Raaga's (diseases).

Paryaya's of Nadi: -

Snayu, Naadi, Hamsi, Dhamani, Dharani, Dharaa, Tantuki, Jivana Gnanaa.

Naadi Pariksha Vidhi:-

The Vaidya Performing Naadi Pariksha should be of:

1. Sthira Chitta
2. Prashantha Atma, Manasaa cha Vishaaradha

Time of Nadi Pariksha:-

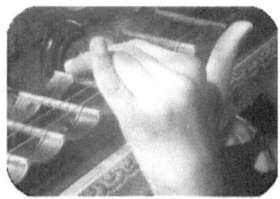

Prabhata kaala.

Positioning of Rogi Hasta:-

While doing Naadi Pariksha, the hand of Rogi is slightly lowered down, with Fingers & Shoulders spreaded, elbow slightly flexed downwards to left, Finger joints are kept free.

The following table tells about holding the Naadi of Rogi:

Vaidya	Purusha Rogi	Stri Rogi
Right Hand is used	Right Hand (pulsations are Predominantly felt)	Left Hand / Left Leg (pulsations are Predominantly felt)
Vaidya should place his 3 fingers in an order as:-	Just below the Angusta Mula	
Tarjani -Index finger– denoting	Vata Dosha in Rogi – Vata Naadi	
Madyama - Middle finger – denoting	Pitta Dosha in Rogi – Pitta Naadi	
Anamika - Ring Finger– denoting	Kapha Dosha in Rogi – Kapha Naadi	

Naadi Pariksha is done 3 times by holding and releasing the hand of Rogi and should be thought over with buddi many times in deciding about the vyadhi.

Naadi Pariksha gives understanding about:-

Dosha involvemnet- v, p, k, vp, vk, pk, vpk.
Condition of 3 doshas
Dosha Gati (Manda, Madyama, Tikshna)
'Dosha Kopa' whether it is Ghana or Alpa.
'Stages of Vyadhi' whether Initial or Final.
Sadya & Asadyata viveka of vyadhi.

Correct assessment is not possible if the Naadi Pariksha is done in following conditions:-

1. Sadyah Snata
2. Sadyah Bhukta
3. Sadyah Sneha
4. Sadyah Avgaahina
5. Kshutaarthi
6. Trushnaarthi
7. Suptasya

Naadi Samsthita Trideva:-

Vaata Naadi	Brahma
Pitta Naadi	Shankara
Kapha Naadi	Vishnu

Naadi Gati:-

Vaata Naadi / Prabanjana Gati	Pitta Naadi / Chapala Gati	Kapha Naadi
Sarpa Gati	Kaka Gati	Raja Hamsa Gati
Jalouka Gati	Laavaka Gati	Mayura Gati
	Manduka Gati	Paravata Kapota Gati
		Kukkuta Gati

Vata Pitta Naadi	Vata Kapha Naadi	Pitta Kapha Naadi	Vata Pitta Kapha Naadi
Muhur Sarpa Gati	Sarpa Gati	Hari Gati	Kashta Kutta-ativega Kuttana Gati
Muhur Manduka Gati	Hamsa Gati	Hamsa Gati	

Nadi if shows any of the following Gati's:	It Indicates:
Gambheera	Mamsa Vahini
Ushna, Vegavati	Jvara vega
Vegavati	Kaama, Krodha
Ksheena	Chinta, Bhaya
Ushna, Gurvi	Rakta Dosha Purna
Gariyasi (weight)	Ama Purna
Laghvi, Vegavati	Deepta agni
Chapala	Kshudita
Sthira	Tripta

Vaatadi Jwara Visesha Suchika Naadi:-					
Vata Jwara	Shita Pitta Jwara	Sleshma Jwara	Vata Pitta Jwara	Vata Kapha Jwara	Pitta Kapha Jwara
Vakra	Dhruta	Manda	Vakra	Ishat Manda	Sukshma
Chapala	Sarala	SuSthira	Ishat Chapala		Shita
Shita Sparsha	Dheerga	Shita	Kathina		Sthira

Lakshanas of Naadi Indicating Health:-

1. Hamsa Naadi
2. Gajagaamini Naadi
3. Prashasta Mukham

The dhamani that is present at the Angusta Mula Bhaaga is **'Jeeva Sakshini Dhamani.'** Its chesta makes understand about the Sukha, Dukha of person.

If the Naadi Pulsates regularly in a rhythmic manner for 30 times at a place, it indicates the person will live for the present time period. If the pulse is otherwise, it indicates 'he may not live' so called as **'Praana Ghatini Naadi.'**(a/c to Vrudda Haarita).

Asadya Naadi Lakshanas: - (indicating Mrityu) / Chikitsa Varjya:-

1. If Pulsates: Mandam Mandam – Shidhilam Shidhilam – Vyakulam Vyakulam & Nityam Skandhe Spurathi.

2. 1st Pulsates with Pitta gati followed by Vata Gati, kapha gati & Chakra Bhramana Gati. Sometimes Bhismatva (Heavy) or Tanautva (thin).
3. Atyanta – Spandana, Kampana & Touches his fingers again & again.

4. Drushyate charane naadi, Kare naiva abidrushyate, Mukham Vikasitam Yasya, Tam Duram parivarjayeth.

5. Vyadhi is Krichra sadya / Asadya if has all the Prakupita 3 Dosha naadi's.

Mrityu occurs	In the Conditions of Naadi & Effects
Within 1 day	Damarukasya Naadi – Thick Pulsations at the Starting & Ending. Thin Pulsations in the Middle.
On 2nd day	Sthira Naadi, some times having Spandana like Vidyut Dhyuti. He lives for 1 day.
On next day	Dosha yukta Naadi, Sheegra, Shitala Naadi.
Within 3 days	Nasthi Mukhe Naadi, Madye Shaityam, Bahih Klama, Manda Naadi.
Within 7 days	Mukhe Naadi vaheth Teevra, Kadachit Sheetala Vaheth, aayati Picchila, sweda.
Within Artha Maasam	Dehe Shaityam, Mukhe Shwasa, Teevra-Vidaaha Naadi.
Gataayu	Ati-Sukshma, Ati-Vega, Shitala Naadi
Akaala Vidyutpaata Iva	Vidyut vat Nimita, Naadi Drusyate/ Na drusyate, Gaccheth Yama Shasanam.

2. Mutra Pariksha:

Just by the knowlwdge of Urine examination the Roga Chihna's gets easily understood.

Mutra Pariksha Vidhi:

Time of performing Pariksha:

Antya Yaama of Nisha (Night). Watch showing 4 am. At that time, Vaidya should wake up Rogi to collect mutra and is kept for examination at Suryodaya. It should be examined many times.

Mutra Grahana:

1. Mutra is collected in a glass vessel.
2. Starting Stream of urine is not to be collected. The later Stream is collected.

Mutra Lakshanas in Vaataadi Dosha:

Vata Dosha	Pitta Dosha	Kapha Dosha	Dwandwaja Dosha	Sannipata Dosha
Panduram	Rakta Varnam	Sa Phenam	Mishrama Varna	Krishna Varna

Mutra Lakshanas in Vaataadi Dosha Prakopa:

Vayu Dosha	Pitta Dosha	Kapha Dosha	Rakta Dosha
Neelam	Peeta	Snigdha	Snigdha
Ruksha	Aruna	Palvala Vaari Tulya (pond water)	Ushna
	Taila Samam		Rakta Varna

Mutra Lakshanas in different conditions:

In the Conditions of:	Mutra Lakshana's:
Ajeerna Prabhava Roga's	Tandula Toya vat Mutra
Nava Jwara	Dhoomra varna, BahuMutram prajayate
Vata Pitta Jwara	Dhoomra Varna, Jalaabham, Ushnam
Vata Kapha Jwara	Shveta Varna, Bhudbudaabam
Pitta Kapha Jwara	Kalusham, Sa Rakta Varna
Jeerna jwara	Asruk sadrisham & Peeta Varna
Sannipata Jwara	Mishra varna

Nagarjuna Kruta Mutra Pariksha:

A Taila Bindu is kept in to the vessel containing urine with help of a Trina (blade of Grass).

Mutra pariksha indicating Sadyata, Kasta sadyata, Asadyata of a Roga.

1. Due to Ati- laghavata of the Mutra, if the Taila Bindu Spreads quickly then the Roga is Sadya.
2. If Don't spread then the Roga is Kasta Sadya.
3. If the Taila Bindu sinks to bottom then the Roga is Asadya.

In a Sadya Vaydhi, if the Taila Bindu Spreads in direction of:			
East	West	North	South
Sheegram Sukhi Baveth	Sukha & Arogya	Gets Cured (Arogita) without Doubt	Jwaram will occur & Arogyam Kramaat Bhaveth

If the Taila Bindu Spreads in direction of:			
Ishanya (N-E)	Agneya (S-E)	Nairuti (S-W)	Vayavya (N-W)
Dies within a Maasa.	Along with spread, if a Chidra happens on the spread then it indicates sure of Mrityu.		The Person Dies even after taking Amrita.

If the taila Bindu Produces any of the following Structures on Mutra, the Rogi should not be considerd for Chikitsa.				
Plough (Halam)	Tortoise (Kurma)	Buffalo (sairibha)	Honey Comb (Karanda Mandala)	Shiro Heena Naram
Gatra Khandam	Shastram	Khadgam	Mushal(Pestle)	Pattisha(Spear with Sharp edge)
Sharam	Dandam	Tri-Chatush Padam		

If the taila Bindu Produces any of the following full Structures on Mutra, the Rogi surely gets treated & Vaidya should proceed for Chikitsa.				
Hamsa	Kaaranda (A type of Duck)	Kamalam	Gaja	Chamara (Yak)
Chatram (Umbrella)	Hamryam (House)	Toranam		

If the Taila Bindu on the mutra Produces:-	It is due to vikriti of:
Sarpa Akaara	Vaata Dosha
Chatra Akaara	Pitta Dosha
Mukta Akaara	Kapha Dosha

If the Taila Bindu on the mutra Produces that which is smililar to:-	It indicates:
Chalini Murti (Sieve Shape)	Kula Dosha certainly
Nara Akaaram (Human form) or	Preta Dosha
Mastaka Dwayam (2 Headed Human)	Bhuta Dosha –>Bhuta Vidya is advised to treat.

By observing the features of Rogi Mutra, the Buddhimaan Vaidya should make a Medication Prescription Internally in his Mind.

3. Mala Pariksha: (as said in RudraTantra.)

Lakshanas of Mala affected with Doshas are as:

Vata Dosha	Pitta Dosha	Kapha Dosha	Sannipata Dosha
Dridata	Peetata	Shuklata	Sarav Lakshana
Sushkata			

Vata Kupita Mala	Vata Kapha Vikara	Vata Pitta Dosha	Pitta Kapha Dosha	Tridosha Vikara
Trutitam	Kapisha Mala	Baddham	Peeta	Shyamam
Phenilam		Su Trutitam	Shwetha	Trutitam
Ruksham		Peeta Shyamam	Ishat Sandram	Peetabham
Dhumalam			Picchilam	Baddha
				Shwetham

Vata Dosha	Pitta Dosha	Kapha Dosha	Ama Malam	Dwandwaja Dosha Malam
Krishanam	Peeta vit	Shwetha varna	Just as kapha Dushita Malam	Mishra Lakshanas
	Kinchit Rakta Varna			

Ajeerna Malam is due to	Swachha Malam is due to
Apakva	Pakva

Jeerna Mala Lakshanas:	Praksheena Mala doshena Dushita Lakshanas:
1. Durgandha	1. Kapila Vrana Varchas
2. Shitala	2. Guti yukta Varchas (pellet like)

Mala Lakshanas in Vyadhi's:		
In Jalodara:	**In Kshaya**	**In Ama Vyadhi's:**
Sitam	Shyama Varna	Peetam
Mahat Malam		Kati vedanam
Puti Gandham		

Roga is Asadya in the following condition of Mala Lakshanas:	
1. Rogi with **Atyagni** passing Mala which is	2. Rogi with **Mandagni** passing Mala which is
Pindita	Dravikruta
Sushka	Durgandha
	Chandrika yukta

Mala Lakshanas indicating Marana	Mala Lakshanas indicating Marana certainly
Ati-Krishna	Ati-Krishna
Ati-Shubra	Ati-Shubra
Ati-Peetam	Ati-Peetam
Arunam	Arunam
	+ Ati-Ushanm

4. Shabdha Pariksha:

Guru Swara indicates	Kapha Dosha
Sphuta Vakta (Clear Voice) indicates	Pitta Dosha
Devoid of Guru & Sphutatva indicates	Vaata Dosha

5. Sparsha Pariksha:

on sparshana if the Rogi is felt as:	It Indicates the Rogi is affected with:
Shitala	Vata Vikara
Ushna	Pitta Vikara
Ardra	Kapahja Vikara

6. Rupa Pariksha:

Among the 3 doshas, Vata is Prabala due to its:	Vata Dosha Manushya Lakshana's:
Vibhutvaat	Doshatmaka (with avaguna's)
AshuKaaritvaat	Kesha & Gatra is of Sphutita & Doosara varna.
Balitvaat	Sheeta Dweshi
Anya kopanaat (provaocate other doshas, dathus etc.)	Chala Dhruti
	Chala Smriti
	Chala Buddhi
Swaatantryaat	Chala Chesta
	Chala Souhaardya(freindship)
Bahu rogatvaat	Chala Drusti
	Chala Gati
	Bahu Pralaapa

Pitta Dosha:	Kapha Dosha:
It is like vahni & its origin is from vahni.	It is like Soma.
Pitta Dosha Udrikta Persons have Lakshana's:	**Kapha dosha Manushya Lakshana's:**
Tikshna Trushna	
Tikshna Bubuksha	Sowmya
Goura Anga	Gooda-Snigdha-Slista→(sandhi-Asthi-Mamsa)
Ushna Anga	
Tamra Hasta Paada Vaktra Anga	not affected by dharma's like: Kshut, Trit, Shoka, Klesha
Shoora (brave)	
Maani (proud)	
Pinga kesha	Buddi yukta
Alpa Roma	Satvika
	Satya Samdha (truth speaking)

7. Drik Pariksha:

Following are Lakshanas present in:

Vata Rogi	Pitta Rogi	Kapha Rogi	Dwandwa dosha Rogi	Tridosha Rogi
Ruksha dristi	Deepa dweshi			Shyama Varna
Dhoomra		Jalaardram drusti	Mishra Lakshana's	Nirbhugnam (looks are straight/ not bent)
Roudra	Santaptam	Jyotisha Hinam	Toornam Toornam Vilochanam (looks are quick)	
Chala				
Antar Jwalati	Peeta Varna	Snigdam		Tandra
		Mandam		Moha
				Roudram
				Rakta Varna

If one of the eye becomes Bhimam (Fearful) & other Militam(closed). Such a Rogi reaches 'Yama Mandira' within 3 days.

If the eyes suddenly becomes jyothi rahita & with Slight Krishna Varna. Such a Rogi move towards 'Yama Shasanam.'

If the dristi preskshana is with Raktam, Krishhna Varna, Roudram. It indicates Mrityu without any samshaya.

If the Dristi of one eye becomes achetana & the taraka (Pupil of eye) is with Bhramana, sphurana, then the Rogi surely follows Paraloka patham (path).

8. Jihwa Pariksha:

Vata Adhikya	Pitta Adhikya	Kapha Adhikya	Tridosha Adhikya	Dwandvaja Adhika
Sheeta	Rakta	Shubra	Krishna	Mishrita Lakshana's
Khara Sparsha	Shyama	Ati Picchila	Kantaka yukta	
Sphutitha			Sushka	

Asya Pariksha:

Vata Rogi	Pitta Rogi	Kapha Rogi	Tridosha Rogi	Ajeerna Rogi	Agnimandya Rogi
Madhura Asyatvam	Katuka Asyata	Madhura Amla Asyata	Sarva Lingam	Ghrita Poorna	Kashaya Asyata

Mrityu Kaala Lakshana's of Manushya:

Sushka Asyam
Shyama Koshta
Asita varna at the biting area of teeth
Sheeta Nasa Pradesha
Shona Aksha Eka Netro (Redness of one eye)
Lulita (unnerved) Kara pada
Stotra Pathitya (loss of/ degradation) Yukta
sometimes Sheeta Shwasa & sometimes Ushna Shwasa
Sheeta gatra prakampa
udvegam
Nishprapancha (no further growth process)

www.ingramcontent.com/pod-product-compliance
Lightning Source LLC
Chambersburg PA
CBHW030950240526
45463CB00016B/2255